The City and the Hospital

The City and the Ocean

The City and the Hospital

The Paradox of Medically Overserved Communities

DANIEL SKINNER,
JONATHAN R. WYNN,
AND BERKELEY FRANZ

The University of Chicago Press
Chicago and London

The University of Chicago Press, Chicago 60637
The University of Chicago Press, Ltd., London
© 2023 by The University of Chicago
Published 2023
Printed and bound by CPI Group (UK) Ltd, Croydon, CR0 4YY

32 31 30 29 28 27 26 25 24 23   1 2 3 4 5

ISBN-13: 978-0-226-82965-4 (cloth)
ISBN-13: 978-0-226-82967-8 (paper)
ISBN-13: 978-0-226-82966-1 (e-book)
DOI: https://doi.org/10.7208/chicago/9780226829661.001.0001

Library of Congress Cataloging-in-Publication Data

Names: Skinner, Daniel, author. | Wynn, Jonathan R., author. |
    Franz, Berkeley A., author.
Title: The city and the hospital : the paradox of medically overserved communities /
    Daniel Skinner, Jonathan R. Wynn, and Berkeley Franz.
Description: Chicago : The University of Chicago Press, 2023. |
    Includes bibliographical references and index.
Identifiers: LCCN 2023008519 | ISBN 9780226829654 (cloth) |
    ISBN 9780226829678 (paperback) | ISBN 9780226829661 (ebook)
Subjects: LCSH: Urban poor—Medical care—United States. | Urban hospitals—
    United States. | Discrimination in medical care—United States.
Classification: LCC RA975.U72 S55 2023 | DDC 362.1086/942—dc23/eng/20230405
LC record available at https://lccn.loc.gov/2023008519

♾ This paper meets the requirements of ANSI/NISO Z39.48-1992 (Permanence of Paper).

Contents

Acronyms

ACA: Affordable Care Act
ACO: Accountable Care Organization
CBO: Community-Based Organization
CDC: Community Development Corporation
CHAT: Community Health Action Team
CHNA: Community Health Needs Assessment
ED: Emergency Department
EMTALA: Emergency Medical Treatment and Labor Act
FQHC: Federally Qualified Health Center
GME: Graduate Medical Education
GUCI: Greater University Circle Initiative (Cleveland)
HHC: Hispanic Health Council (Hartford)
HRSA: Health Resources and Services Administration
IRS: Internal Revenue Service
MUA/P: Medically Underserved Areas/Populations
SINA: Southside Institutions Neighborhood Alliance (Hartford)

Introduction

A hospital/medical center can no longer think of itself as an island, or for whatever reasons exempt from its urban ecological context . . . To "do no harm" now denotes far more than it did a century or even a mere decade ago: a hospital must cause neither human nor ecological harm.

STEPHEN VERDERBER, *Innovations in Hospital Architecture*[1]

A Billion-Dollar Question

In the historic Hough neighborhood of Cleveland, Ohio, just blocks from stretches of old brownstones peppered with empty lots, sits the main campus of the world-renowned Cleveland Clinic. The sprawling, ever-expanding, and undeniably impressive mega-complex is the birthplace of some of the world's most important medical innovations as well as home to top-ranked providers in cardiac care and other specialties. In the shadow of the Clinic's world-class facilities, we interviewed Janey, the head of a local nonprofit, in her nondescript office.[2] When we asked her how hospitals could improve their relationships with the surrounding communities, she said with a sigh, "That is a tough question," and then added, "Actually, that's the million-dollar question." What Janey referred to as a "million-dollar question" is the primary focus of this book. It is, in fact, a billion-dollar question.

The question of how to improve hospital/community relationships can be framed by a paradox. Most U.S. city skylines contain at least one noticeable hospital tower. Those looming spires—buffered by an array of administrative buildings, specialty centers, parking garages, and even hotels—are also invisibly linked to regional and even national hospital and healthcare systems. On the surface, it appears that healthcare services would be easily accessible to most urbanites, and hospitals are straightforward assets for urban communities. Yet the U.S. Health Resources and Services Administration (HRSA) classifies many of the neighborhoods—often primarily communities of color—just beyond the doors of urban hospitals as "medically underserved," meaning they have "too few primary care providers, high infant mortality, high poverty or a high elderly population."[3] Indeed, in many U.S. cities, residents living mere blocks from top-ranked healthcare institutions face severe "economic, linguistic, or cultural barriers to healthcare."[4] How can residents sitting in the shadow of an elite healthcare institution have such difficulty obtaining adequate healthcare?

In many of these communities, industries and retail have long since moved to the suburbs, leaving widespread income and wealth inequality in their ebbing tide. Hospitals are referred to as "anchor institutions" for a reason.[5] Although some urban hospitals relocate, they are less likely than other institutions to leave their home neighborhoods. This pattern creates an unlikely pairing of highly resourced institutions providing healthcare services to the broader city, state, and region, on one hand, and disinvested neighborhoods whose residents face profound social and economic barriers to maintaining good health, on the other.[6] For example, the Fairfax neighborhood near the Cleveland Clinic has a disproportionately high level of chronic disease. This dynamic is not lost on the neighborhood residents and public health advocates we interviewed. As Aundra, a former Cleveland resident, lamented: "The people in the community have really suffered, and they're still suffering . . . The Clinic is just in such close proximity and could help them so much. They're not doing it. So, I mean, great medical care is within reach of these people and they're just not getting it. That's not fair."

We call the scenario Aundra described—high-end medical institutions located in economically distressed communities with poor health outcomes— the "paradox of medically-overserved communities." This play on the HRSA designation of "underserved" communities captures the fact that, if one were to look at their resources on a map, we would expect these communities to be among the most medically "overserved" areas in the U.S. The paradox is created by the fact that the presence of throngs of healthcare professionals and expensive healthcare facilities somehow fails to improve the health of those communities in the ways we would expect. Indeed, in some cases we find evidence that these hospitals may make the health of their communities worse, not because of anything concerning direct medical services, but for reasons owing to their presence as a large urban institution that makes daily decisions that affect the community.

The answers needed to understand this paradox are both obvious and complicated. In the post-war period of heavy white and capital flight, cities lost major employers and institutions to outlying areas, and city planners and residents turned to emplaced institutions to rethink and develop their missions and engage their communities in economic development and health improvement. In addition, growing awareness of inequality broadly and persistent patterns of health disparities that disproportionately impact marginalized groups increasingly shape the expectations communities have of their institutions. While these institutions, including hospitals, have the potential to play a key role in the present and future of the nation's cities, the motivation and commit-ment to enact meaningful change remain uneven and ambiguous. However, researchers, city planners, and residents are beginning to reach a consensus around the importance of providing community health as a way to both re-duce costs for individuals and healthcare providers and create the precondi-tions necessary to improve health outcomes and reduce health inequities.

Given these geographical and institutional conditions, contemporary con-versations about healthcare and community health are ripe for discussions about what hospitals can and should do for their neighborhoods. There is an urgent need for dialogue between multiple stakeholders including healthcare practitioners and administrators; researchers in the fields of public policy, ur-ban sociology, and political science; city planners; and engaged citizens. This book aims to provide critical information for that conversation.

Putting Health Disparities in Place

Contemporary claims of a new "placeless" society obscure the tangible, mate-rial factors that shape neighborhoods and their residents. Recent studies of cities show that "neighborhood effects" continue to influence a variety of out-comes, including health.[7] Exploring what he called "the new urban question," and while acknowledging the importance of larger economic and political trends, Robert Sampson posited that neighborhood context generates much of the socioeconomic inequality found in cities.[8] Both socioeconomic inequal-ity and other factors, especially racism, underlie the relationship between neigh-borhood context and health outcomes. The focus of this book is on the gaps that exist between social groups when it comes to health outcomes such as life expectancy and chronic disease rates. These health disparities are not the result of fixed biological or genetic differences between groups but are shaped by social factors, especially patterns of social inequality and pathways for so-cial mobility that are deeply ingrained in the neighborhood context. Neigh-borhood effects on health are perhaps so influential that they've led research-ers and practitioners in the fields of healthcare and public health to emphasize that zip codes, not genetic codes, are what shape health outcomes.[9] Even zip codes, however, may not capture the fact that health outcomes can shift from block to block, depending on factors such as the quality of housing and the proximity of nearby economic, educational, or healthcare institutions. Some-times these institutions are directly across the street (see fig. 0.1).

Given the firm emplacement of health disparities in U.S. cities, there is an urgent need to identify sources of durable investment in neglected and actively disadvantaged urban communities that are disproportionately populated by residents of color.[10] By examining the relationship between the hospital and the surrounding communities, this book identifies important neighborhood effects and shows how hospitals can influence these effects, either exacerbating or reducing socioeconomic and racial inequalities and, by extension, health outcomes. We view hospitals as important urban institutions that play a central role in answering this new urban question of neighborhood effects.

Hospitals have been a significant part of Americans' social lives for over a century. Fully 99 percent of Americans are born in hospitals, and people die in hospitals at slightly greater rates than at home[11]—although during the pandemic, COVID-related deaths were far more likely to occur at the hospital than at home, with rates differing based on age and race/ethnicity.[12] The American Hospital Association identified 6,093 U.S. hospitals in their 2022 annual census of hospitals. Most of these (5,139) were community as opposed to specialty hospitals, including 2,960 private not-for-profit hospitals, 1,228 investor-owned or for-profit hospitals, and 951 public hospitals.[13] In the case of the University of Colorado Hospital, the public, nonprofit hospital featured in this book, its classification does not have significant consequences in terms of how it is operated; indeed, our interviewees did not even mention the hospital's legal status in interviews.[14] In contrast, one distinction that does have significant repercussions for hospitals is urban versus suburban/rural location.

Like other anchor institutions (e.g., universities, art and cultural facilities, libraries, sports facilities, school districts, and other major employers), hospitals can forge collaborative and productive relationships with surrounding communities and their residents—for example, they can generate positive memories of the birth of a child or the relief offered by a surgery.[15] And, just like other city institutions, hospitals can also prompt feelings of disappointment, anger, and frustration. Many well-known institutions have historically acrimonious relationships with their neighbors, and while some of these institutions have begun to take steps to remedy these histories, the work is often slow and challenging, with uneven results.[16] Davarian Baldwin's book *In the Shadow of the Ivory Tower* illustrates this type of troubled history by recounting Johns Hopkins University's displacement of 742 Black families to make way for a biotech park, a development that shows how urban academic institutions promote and perhaps overstate their economic impact while simultaneously hiding their hand in the perpetuation of deeper inequities, particularly among poorer and non-white communities.[17] In conversations about the relationships between cities and institutions, so-called Eds and Meds (universities and healthcare organizations) are distinct from other institutions because of their explicit missions of providing education and care. For the

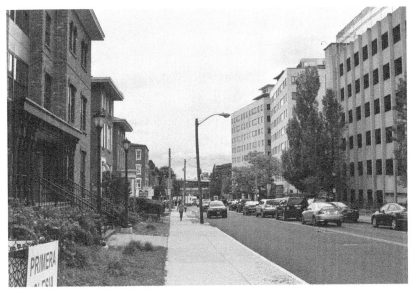

FIGURE 0.1. Looking east on Jefferson Street, Hartford Hospital on the right and buildings that were purchased by the hospital on the left (Photo by Wynn)

"Meds," which are concerned with health outcomes and community well-being, this means being subject to a unique set of expectations regarding care provision. What it means to provide care, however, is subject to much debate.

In Cleveland, we met Mansfield Frazier. Until his death in 2021, Frazier was the executive director of Neighborhood Solutions, an organization focused on job creation and community revitalization, achieved primarily through re-purposing vacant lots for urban farming projects. He was also a vintner who took great pride in his vineyards in the heart of the Hough neighborhood on the east side of Cleveland near the Clinic's main campus. Frazier, who had once been incarcerated on a charge of counterfeiting credit cards, used the winery, which he called Château Hough, to support his efforts to help formerly in-carcerated individuals reenter society. During our conversation, he joked that the wine made at Château Hough had a special terroir because the grapes were grown on land that used to house a crack cocaine operation.

In our conversation, Frazier discussed a shift in how hospitals and institutions of higher education located in urban areas perceived their relationship with the surrounding communities: "Thirty, thirty-five years ago, places like Brown University, Temple University, they were in the middle of Black communities, and so was Case Western and the Cleveland Clinic, so somebody at those universities said, 'Wait a minute, we're building walls; we've been build-ing walls to the larger community instead of bridges.' So, they started changing

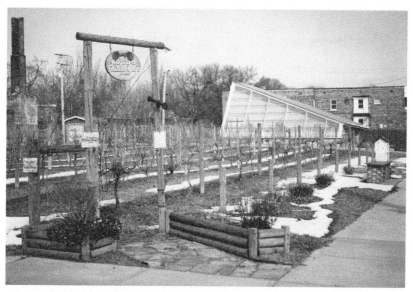

FIGURE 0.2. Mansfield Frazier's Château Hough Vineyards, on Hough Avenue and East 66th Street (Photo by Mark Franz)

their outlook on how they were interacting with their neighborhoods. Cleveland Clinic and University Circle were very late to the dance."

While a poor attribute on the dance floor, fixity is one of the key factors underlying the neighborhood relationships of anchor institutions like universities and hospitals. Their "anchor" status means that hospitals can serve as potential sites of connection and coordination at both the individual and, increasingly, citywide levels, particularly as municipalities look to these organizations when strategizing how to stabilize urban economies and communities. When discussing Hartford's transformation from the home of a stable and locally invested multibillion-dollar insurance industry in the mid-twentieth century to a city with a revolving series of CEOs and evaporating industry, a local community leader commented that "the hospitals have withstood the test of time." And yet, relative permanence can be a double-edged sword. Anchors can do an enormous amount of good for communities, but they are well positioned to do long-term harm as well—a point with clear Hippocratic resonance, as the chapter's epigraph suggests.

If institutions opt to engage communities in an intentional and careful manner, they can use their ample power to improve health and social outcomes in local neighborhoods. Yet even if there were consensus on how hospitals can or should improve community health—and this book makes clear that there isn't—hospitals are ill prepared for the enormity of the task. Ready or not, how-ever, some communities have forced these powerful and cloistered institu-tions to become more responsive to their needs, frequently in the aftermath of an animating event that created public relations problems.

At the same time, hospitals and medical centers leverage their workforce and health access narratives to extract maximally beneficial situations for themselves. If they cannot alter situations to their advantage, hospitals may consider relocating. This was the case with the University of Colorado Hos-pital, which moved six miles east, from downtown Denver to Aurora, in 2007. Similarly, after decades in the long-struggling westside Columbus, Ohio, neigh-borhood of Franklinton, the Mt. Carmel Health System relocated its main hospital to the affluent suburb of Grove City, leaving the community without a major healthcare anchor.[18] Likewise, the Texas Medical Center moved be-yond Houston's city limits to capitalize on cheaper and more abundant space, building new facilities and attracting not only new staff and patients, but enough hotels, restaurants, and other services to now be known as a "medi-cal city"—a name that is enshrined in the for-profit healthcare system that dominates the area, Medical City Healthcare.[19] Other hospitals may want to relocate but find it impractical to do so. Richard, a nonprofit executive who works closely with U.S. hospitals and other institutions on community devel-opment, explained that it is difficult for anchors to move. He concluded that regardless of whether they are nonprofit, after 50-plus years of urban disin-vestment and white flight, many hospitals have "probably considered [leav-ing], but maybe it was too expensive to pick up their entire infrastructure and move it to the suburbs." At a minimum, the movement and consolida-tion of medical institutions into cloistered sites is an ongoing urban—and suburban—phenomenon.

While major corporations and anchors once served as paternalistic forces within many cities, globalization and capital flight have shaken the economic and social well-being of many urban neighborhoods. These trends left medi-cal institutions—which are tangible components of regional healthcare mega-corporations and constitute a significant slice of municipal economic health[20]—in the position of serving as stewards of qualitatively different work than that encapsulated in their mission statements. At the same time, these institutions can serve as intractable forces of harm if they neglect community health, or exhibit indifference to or even hostility toward community needs and val-ues.[21] This urban complexity raises two primary questions about the hospital and the city: What is a hospital's responsibility to surrounding communities, and how can communities and hospitals work together?

Examining Healthcare in the City

The impetus for this collaboration was a two-pronged assessment of recent developments in the healthcare landscape: we sensed that provisions in the Affordable Care Act (ACA) requiring hospitals to engage in community-oriented work were a promising answer to the growing call to improve population health and reduce health disparities, but we were uncertain about how hospitals would respond to these new reporting requirements and whether their actions would generate meaningful improvements in health outcomes. Beyond the ACA, state and local municipalities have increasingly sought to leverage anchor institutions such as hospitals to improve local communities, although these efforts have met with mixed success.[22] This situation presented the opportunity to examine hospitals and urban neighborhoods in order to understand the current scenario and, perhaps more importantly, the potential for even better outcomes.

There is, of course, a wealth of research on both community health and hospitals.[23] Urban sociology, however, tends to overlook hospitals, just as medical literature has for too long tended to overlook the community health orientation of healthcare institutions.[24] Yet the relationship between hospital and community is an illuminating story of opportunity, inequity, and racialized spaces and institutions.[25] Even the most casual of observers will note that urban hospitals are often located in low-income and poorly represented communities. Most urban hospitals provide emergency services and trauma care for the racially and ethnically diverse communities that surround them—many of whom are uninsured, underinsured, or Medicaid recipients—indeed, they are required to do so by law,[26] but the provision of routine healthcare to the local population largely falls to a "dedicated but frequently fragmented and financially fragile" safety net of public hospitals, community health centers, clinics, and health departments.[27] In most cases, the key point of contact between hospitals and communities are emergency departments with their dreary waiting rooms, where patients are cared for but discharged as quickly as possible. While recent critiques of U.S. healthcare have focused on the overuse of medical services, in truth, hospitals are, for many, places to be avoided.[28]

Meanwhile, deeper inside the boundaries of the modern urban hospital campus reside billion-dollar medical devices used for groundbreaking treatments—ranging from robot-assisted surgery to diagnostic procedures conducted with next-generation imaging systems—as well as a wide and growing range of artificial intelligence technologies capable of futuristic machine learning. When we toured the Cleveland Clinic, for example, we saw impressive examples of high-tech medical equipment, including a fully computer-

ized endoscopy lab, which places the Clinic at the forefront of urologic lapa-
roscopic and robotic surgery. Our tour guide was eager to show us one of
the 12 VIP suites where the Clinic's affluent and famous patients have stayed,
including, among others, Oprah Winfrey, Robin Williams, Saudi princes, professional athletes, and world leaders.[29] We also saw the Clinic's remarkable
subterranean corridors where robots confidently mingle—seamlessly though
cautiously—with human employees, delivering soiled linens for cleaning, han-
dling mail, and performing a wide range of other tasks.

Toward the end of the tour, the guide ushered us into the Rooftop Pavilion
in the Clinic's newest and most recognizable building, where we enjoyed a
10th-floor view of the campus and the neighborhoods just beyond its borders.
As we scanned the impressive view, looking west along Euclid Avenue toward
the skyline of downtown Cleveland, and then, much closer, to the Hough neighborhood to the north and the Fairfax neighborhood to the south, the tour
guide called our attention to one of the Clinic's key competitors—University
Hospitals—which was visible through a southeast-facing window. The modern, high-tech facilities beneath our feet stood in sharp contrast to the buildings and property in these nearby communities.

The stark difference between the services offered to princes and movie stars
and those offered to average Clevelanders belies the idea that these institutions aim to serve communities in an equitable manner. Despite these disparities, hospitals and communities remain deeply entwined. Beyond the large,
imposing structures of hospitals with their well-heeled physician groups, there
are rolling healthcare clinics, medical interpreters, and a host of other people
and places that comprise the broader system of healthcare. Hospitals, as shown
throughout this book, do much more than provide medical services. For example, a hospital might help support a neighborhood farmers market, hire
local residents, source materials from local businesses, and stabilize neighborhood housing stock. At the same time, hospitals may negatively, if inadver-
tently, impact communities as they expand, shape, and overtake surrounding
neighborhoods.

An Integrated Approach to Hospitals and Cities

This book arrives at a time of broad institutional change and in the wake of
a global pandemic that raised new and important questions about healthcare
and rekindled long-standing concerns. The research herein aims to clarify the
contours of these changes. It is likely, however, that the current stage of this
transition will persist for some time. Barring an unprecedented (and in many
ways unimaginable) technological revolution in medicine, hospitals will

remain formidable and comparatively stable urban facilities well into the future. Unlocking their potential as centers for not just health, but urban life more broadly, could radically change cities. Such a transformation would also leverage the significant potential these institutions have to improve population health and reduce health inequalities. Imagine, for a moment, hospitals taking a cue from libraries and becoming places for public gathering and connection, wherein health professionals and members of the community engage with one another—in other words, becoming "palaces for the people"[30] instead of either cloisters for elites or isolated spaces for the underserved. What would this new type of hospital look like?

There are a few frameworks that suggest answers to this question. Anthropologist Arthur Kleinman described care as an embodied experience—a series of physical acts of "touching, embracing, steadying, lifting, toileting," as well as the tone of voice, the gaze, and simple presence.[31] Such care is relational and reciprocal. Could this approach be applied to the relationship between hospitals and their communities? Can researchers and stakeholders understand this partnership as a series of interactions that comprise care? To be sure, the idea of "social determinants of health" is widely known and increasingly discussed among healthcare professionals. Some hospitals already address, sometimes quite actively, social determinants in their neighborhoods. And yet, some visions—from both hospitals and community members—of what a new type of hospital would look like seem to only add to the long list of one-off or forgotten initiatives, rather than engendering a structural shift toward greater collaboration and transparency with communities, as well as broader definitions of community benefit and population health.

When re-envisioning the hospital/community relationship in urban areas, there is a danger of inappropriately medicalizing urban communities. We are not advocating for a narrowly focused expansion of traditional biomedical approaches that tend to overlook the social causes of disease and the social implications of medical care. Rather, meaningful advancements in healthcare entail new modes of engagement with individuals and call for both the infusion of new funds into community-directed initiatives as well as a qualitative shift in the allocation of resources. This mode of engagement requires hospitals and medical centers to interact with surrounding communities in a collaborative, historically informed, and ethical manner.[32] Thus, this book explores how hospitals can become true community-focused entities not by medicalizing and controlling the local community, but by collaborating with the community to improve health outcomes and reduce social inequality.

Finally, this project is an attempt to examine the wider structural, systematic, and even geographic factors producing healthcare inequalities, with a focus on hospitals and medical centers. The book, therefore, centers on potential strategies and solutions that transcend hospital walls and campuses. We argue that it is in these solutions and strategies, and in the oft-overlooked spaces in hospital/community relationships, that the city and the hospital can discover the next stage of co-existence and collaboration.

Our Cases and the Outline for the Book

To understand how urban healthcare institutions interact with their communities, we explored the dynamics of power, history, race, and urbanity as much as the workings of the medical field. Building on prior quantitative studies and policy briefs focused on anchor institutions,[33] as well as qualitative studies examining how hospitals and healthcare facilities interact with local communities,[34] this book pursues a multidimensional analysis of the hospital/community relationship, including examinations of large-scale structural changes (e.g., urban redevelopment initiatives and changes in healthcare policy), meso-level changes (e.g., the development of new institutional roles), and micro-level changes (e.g., shifts in individual meanings and values).

The City and the Hospital[35] is grounded in case studies of three urban hospitals: Hartford Hospital in Hartford, Connecticut; the Cleveland Clinic in Cleveland, Ohio; and the University of Colorado Hospital, located on the larger Anschutz Medical Campus in Aurora, Colorado. Although some characteristics unite these three hospitals (see table 0.1), they operate in different regions of the country and in unique communities, and each institution faces specific challenges and opportunities both inside and beyond the campus perimeters. Hartford Hospital, the crown jewel of the Hartford HealthCare system, was established over a century ago and has served the needs of the city to varying degrees since that time. Like many other U.S. hospitals, it has sought to become a destination for healthcare in the region and the country. The Cleveland Clinic has collaborated with other anchor institutions via the "University Circle Partnership," yet the main campus focuses on providing specialty care, which raises a host of questions about what should be expected of such an institution, especially given its location in two high-need communities. The third hospital, the University of Colorado Hospital, offers a rare example of an anchor institution that moved out of an urban area, in this case from downtown Denver to Aurora, and subsequently forged new community relationships and developed new community service goals.

Two of our cases, the Cleveland Clinic and Hartford Hospital, are predominantly private nonprofit entities, classified by the IRS as 501(c)(3) "charitable" organizations, and thus must balance the need to secure their futures as

TABLE 0.1. Hospital and community characteristics across three cases

	Hartford Hospital	Cleveland Clinic	University of Colorado Hospital
Staffed beds	927	1,325	665
Control type	Private, nonprofit	Private, nonprofit	Government
Teaching status	Major	Major	Major
Number of residents/interns	247	908	454
Total annual patient revenue	$4,010,638,314	$16,959,307,334	$10,290,754,324
Trauma status	Level 1	Non-trauma center	Level 1
Region	Northeast	Midwest	West
Percent of children in poverty	14%	24%	12%
County unemployment rate	3.9%	4.2%	2.9%

Source: American Hospital Directory; County Health Rankings and Roadmaps Report 2021.

private, revenue-dependent entities with their efforts to improve community health in exchange for tax exemption. The University of Colorado Hospital, in contrast, is part of the University of Colorado Hospital Authority, an organization affiliated with the state government, as well as the broader University of Colorado Anschutz Medical Campus, a complex of hospitals and medical education facilities.

In addition to examining the differences between these hospitals and their respective communities, we explored the diversity of thought within them. Neither "the hospital" nor "the community" is a monolith. Both are aggregates of various cultures and positions that overlap and intersect in meaningful ways. As such, we are careful not to overgeneralize about a specific hospital's mission or work and highlight different perspectives within each institution.

Our aim was to use our data to draw comparisons and establish connections across a variety of cases to contribute to our understanding of urban health. Capturing the connections and comparisons across these cases was the central motivation for our conducting more than 200 interviews with hospital administrators and employees, community-based organization leaders, real estate brokers, local business owners, foundation presidents, food activists, police, university campus administrators, government representatives, and members of the community, in their houses and in local businesses (see Appendix A).

Two important dynamics are worth noting. First, hospital administrators were, unsurprisingly, cautious about speaking with us. Like executives in most large organizations, hospital executives are allergic to negative public relations and likely dissuade employees from media appearances. Given this mindset, we were provided what we would characterize as fair access to "upper-middle-level" people in these organizations: we interviewed high-level physicians and administrators on all three campuses. It took months to gain the trust of key players and access to these institutions—our status as university professors likely influenced our ability to eventually succeed—and the facilities and interviewees we had access to tended to be highly curated, although this level of attention was more exacting at some institutions (especially the Cleveland Clinic) than others. Second, while community members often had pointed criticisms they wished to share with us, they were at times understandably cautious of three white researchers entering their predominantly non-white communities and asking questions about local health outcomes and community perceptions of institutions. Obtaining a full and accurate view of the hospital/city relationship required the research team to be persistent and strategic in our interviewee selection. We expand on these issues and explain the study design, data collection, and use of pseudonyms and real names in Appendix A: On Methods.

The interview data provide an important snapshot of perceptions among community members and other stakeholders, and thus shed light on the contexts and perspectives that serve as the backdrop for hospital/community relations. The arc of the book reveals a compelling account that recasts urban hospitals in a new light—as not only medical institutions in the traditional sense, but also a complex urban force.

Chapter 1 provides the context for answering a basic but crucial question: Why are so many communities surrounding hospital campuses in such a precarious state of health? This chapter presents quantitative data and community perspectives on health disparities and examines traditional assumptions about how hospitals and communities coexist as well as how both experience and contribute to the health inequality that persists in many major U.S. cities. This chapter also introduces the three case studies, using health outcomes and disparities as a framework for understanding how each case is uniquely situated within a broader social and economic context.

Chapter 2 looks to local histories and community memories to understand current health challenges and relationships between the three hospitals and their respective communities. We explore how local histories and contentious terms (place, community, and access) have been contested and changed over time, binding and challenging the fragile relationship between institution and neighborhood.

Chapter 3 illustrates how hospitals engage in community development. First, we examine what we call the hospitals' "explicit community development agendas," which comprise the formal programs and initiatives the hospitals use to engage with their communities. These strategies tend to cohere around hire local, live local, and buy local programs, which many hospitals undertake, although with mixed results. The second half of the chapter details the hospitals' "implicit community agendas," which include efforts to secure neighboring properties and develop innovation corridors, actions contributing to gentrification and displacement.

In chapter 4, we draw on the concept of a "contact zone" to discuss the places hospitals and communities meet, including points of friction, conflicts, and collaborations. These sites function in complex and often contradictory ways. Against this backdrop, we discuss experiences with medical care—good and bad—in the context of larger structural issues that produce asymmetries, shift boundaries, and offer opportunities, often along racial, ethnic, and class lines.

Chapter 5 provides an overview of the broad categories both professionals and residents use to construct their expectations of medical institutions. In providing a taxonomy of these expectations, we argue that each type has distinct implications for the development of and advocacy for policies that could reshape how researchers, stakeholders, and policymakers think about hospitals and communities. This chapter shows that several types of expectations—differing in both quality and intensity—coexist within these neighborhoods and even within the hospital campuses themselves.

Finally, the conclusion offers a brief outline of the existing policies that shape hospital/community interaction and highlights six policy proposals that can contribute to urban population health. We approach policy expansively here, including internal strategies related to the design and use of space within hospitals and medical centers. The uneven developments we describe throughout the book, which we argue will become increasingly common, underscore this chapter's arguments. Accordingly, our approach to the future assumes that hospitals and communities will continue to engage one another in ways that could yield short-term policy change, even as long-term policy changes begin to unfold.

Overall, this book is a collaboration between a political scientist (Skinner), an urban and cultural sociologist (Wynn), and a medical sociologist (Franz) who brought different skill sets and scholarly lenses to the project. We developed this book over nearly six years, and our contributions to the final product varied according to each individual's expertise, availability, and career course. Skinner and Wynn conceptualized the study and share first authorship. Skinner and Franz conducted the bulk of the interviews in Cleveland and Aurora, while Wynn conducted the bulk of the interviews in Hartford. Franz and Skinner received funding to support research travel and participant incentives. Franz coordinated with Ohio University's Institutional Review Board, as Wynn did with the research review office at the University of Massachusetts Amherst. Franz contributed early drafts of chapters 1 and 2, including secondary data analysis and tables/figures, made substantive additions to those chapters afterward, and contributed suggestions and edits to the rest of the manuscript. Wynn led on early drafts of chapters 2, 3, and 4, and Skinner led early drafts of chapters 5 and 6. Skinner and Wynn co-led writing the introduction and Appendix A: On Methods, and completed the majority of editing, restructuring, and final preparation of the manuscript.

An Opportunity for Transformation

U.S. hospitals evolved from places where patients went to die to places of recovery and restoration. They also evolved from places primarily serving the poor, to Janus-faced institutions seeking to treat their local communities while increasingly looking to attract well-heeled patients through state-of-the-art medical procedures. Hospitals will undoubtedly continue to evolve, and the questions we consider in this book concern the next, as-yet-unwritten, chapter of the urban hospital. We believe the current scenario offers an opportunity to compel hospitals to assume new and innovative roles in improving the health of communities. The resultant image of the hospital as an urban institution is a valuable contribution to conversations between healthcare providers, urban communities, and policymakers who seek to improve the relationship between healthcare anchor institutions and their neighbors. We hope the book will allow readers to see hospitals, communities, and the hospital/community dynamic through fresh eyes. New modes of thought about institutions create new expectations, which in turn transform these institutions and the dynamics surrounding them.

At the center of these discussions is the question of whether hospitals will adjust their traditional roles as sites for medical education and clinical care by increasingly addressing public health and neighborhood well-being. As we show, however, such a shift requires hospitals and, importantly, communities to address multiple deep-seated issues and dynamics. While we cannot predict exactly how the hospital/city relationship will evolve, this book takes an important step toward understanding the current situation by identifying and describing the key stakeholders, processes, and spaces that shape the relationship between urban hospitals and communities.

1

Why Are So Many Hospital Neighborhoods Health Poor?

How you could reconcile the health of the population against some of the really incredible resources that are so close at hand is something that we . . . work on every day.
PERSIS SOSIAK, former Commissioner of Health, Cleveland
Department of Public Health

Contrasts are easy to spot when walking around Hartford Hospital's campus. Standing at the southern border, at the corner of Washington Street and Retreat Avenue, a visitor can see the Learning Corridor, a knot of four magnet schools sitting on land purchased and developed in collaboration with a community organization funded by the hospital, nearby Trinity College, and other downtown institutions. In one direction is a mural reading "El Monumento a la Familia Puertorriqueña," with the explanation "Honoring the contribution of the Puerto Rican families to the development of the United States of America." In another direction is the Institute of Living, a psychiatric hospital acquired by Hartford Hospital in 1994. The Institute's central tower is adorned not by the rod of Asclepius (which represents the god of healing), but rather by the caduceus: the winged staff, with two entwined serpents, of Hermes—the god of merchants and thieves, and the messenger of the dead. This mistaken but telling symbolism is common in American healthcare.[1]

Pedestrians have a choice. If they walk north on Washington Street, they enter the lively and predominantly Puerto Rican community of Frog Hollow, a historic district (as designated by the National Register of Historic Places) due to its rich industrial history, active community planning, and the Victorian homes that stand as noble reminders of its industrial heyday. Today, however, the area is one of the state's poorest zip codes and is a Medically Underserved Area. Pedestrians who choose to walk up Retreat Avenue enter a campus of buildings, each emblazoned with a logo consisting of multicolored quotation marks, signifying the Hartford HealthCare system, of which Hartford Hospital has long been the flagship facility. Rising above the tree line is the sparkling new $150 million Bone and Joint Institute, which caters to a decidedly non-local clientele. The institute is geared toward capturing a growing national market of wealthy baby boomers with aging knees and ankles. Its sweeping ribbons of white and reflective glass stretch across Retreat Avenue.

While stark and perhaps surprising, vast inequality is common among urban hospital landscapes like Hartford's. Life expectancy in the U.S. has effectively doubled over the last century. The Kaiser Family Foundation, however, estimates that lack of access to formal healthcare services accounts for only about 10 percent of premature deaths in the U.S.[2] With the exception of paradigm-changing drugs such as statins and penicillin, advancements in areas such as sanitation, along with health promotion efforts such as vaccination campaigns and tobacco cessation education, have been much more powerful drivers of health and well-being.[3] Yet public health spending lags far behind medical care expenditures. Misaligned priorities in focus and funding have resulted in increasingly poor health outcomes in the U.S. relative to other industrialized countries.[4]

Mirroring wider economic and social inequalities in the U.S., good health— from infant mortality to life expectancy—is highly stratified. A growing field of research focuses on the social factors shaping health outcomes, broadly referred to as "social and structural determinants of health." This phrase refers to so-called upstream social factors such as economic security, housing, education, and unemployment, which, in combination with healthcare access, largely shape the health of individuals and more importantly create gaps or disparities within communities and populations.[5] Above all, studies aiming to uncover the social determinants of health emphasize the mechanisms by which material and social resources shape health outcomes and improve social conditions.[6]

A Latina Hartfordite who works in community health centers described the health disparities she sees in her neighborhoods: "We know that people in Hartford have a disproportionate level of diabetes, asthma, and hypertension. And part of the asthma issue, we think, has to do with the older housing stock. I think there's a lot of theories out there about why asthma is so much higher in certain areas, pockets. Do geo-mapping of where asthma is very prevalent. Hartford has many neighborhoods where it would show bright red on that map, and it's usually tied to old housing stock." Indeed, while interior factors of quality housing affect health (e.g., lead paint and mold inside a home exacerbate asthma), the location of a home determines health as well.[7] Location factors include proximity to environmental hazards and subsequent air quality, and the absence of social and safe outdoor spaces may predispose a community to crime, preclude opportunities to exercise, and erode social cohesion.[8]

Housing is only one factor. Limited job opportunities and systemic racism in educational and economic institutions also curb social mobility, contribute to chronic stress, and limit healthcare access through employer-based insurance programs.[9] Historical real estate practices, especially those that promoted and maintained residential segregation,[10] prevented many Americans, especially Black Americans, from accumulating wealth, and these same neighborhoods are increasingly likely to experience high levels of chronic illness and premature death. A major longitudinal study of cardiac outcomes among Americans found that when residents of highly segregated neighborhoods moved into less segregated neighborhoods, their blood pressure readings measurably decreased.[11] In major U.S. cities, residents in disadvantaged neighborhoods die much younger, sometimes by as much as 25 years, than their counterparts in more affluent neighborhoods.[12] Life expectancy in Chicago, for example, can rise and fall by 15–30 years across the distance of just a mile or two.[13] These trends have become of such interest to policymakers, public health practitioners, and local activists that researchers have created interactive tools for comparing neighborhoods, such as the "City Health Dashboard" supported by the NYU School of Medicine.[14]

Evidence like this prompted well-known physician and author Abraham Verghese to declare that geography is "destiny," which has since become conventional wisdom in the scholarly community health literature.[15] Indeed, many researchers and healthcare professionals have similarly brought focus to environmental and neighborhood factors as shaping the most intimate details of Americans' lives, how long we live and what quality of health we can expect while we're alive. In a major shift from the decades-long emphasis on genomics and precision medicine, many healthcare and public health leaders now agree that social factors should be the focus of interventions to improve the health of communities. Some large healthcare institutions that once focused on treating sick patients are now taking steps to address these upstream factors in hopes of preventing costly-to-treat illnesses and improving overall health outcomes.[16] Clearly, urban hospitals, which receive a substantial proportion of healthcare funding, must be part of the solution. The questions are how, and to what degree?

Hospitals and Community Health

If healthcare services truly shaped health outcomes, we could expect living close to a well-regarded hospital to be a strong predictor of good health. After all, lifesaving care at a major medical center would be only a short walk or quick drive away in the event of an emergency. But would such proximity reduce, prevent, or delay some of the leading causes of death in the U.S., such as heart disease, cancer, or chronic respiratory conditions? Residential proximity to a medical center, it turns out, is a more complicated story.[17]

Given that increases in life expectancy over the last century were not experienced equally across racial, ethnic, and socioeconomic groups, these dynamics should not be surprising. They do, however, reveal an erroneous assumption. Even when communities reside in the shadow of large, powerful, and well-capitalized medical institutions, they can be technically designated as "medically underserved." One in five U.S. private nonprofit hospitals are in high-poverty, urban neighborhoods, and many of the top-ranked U.S. medical centers (regardless of ownership status) straddle extremely health-poor neighborhoods.[18]

Nationally available data show that among the top-ranked hospitals in the U.S., those with the most profound disparities include the Mayo Clinic's Jacksonville, Florida, campus, where the percentage of locals older than 18 with cancer is 89.73 percent greater than the citywide average. In the area surrounding the University of Michigan Hospital, the percentage of residents missing all their teeth is 152.81 percent greater than the citywide average. Similarly, outside the University of Southern California's Keck Hospital, in Los Angeles, the percentage of residents without access to health insurance is 71.26 percent greater than the citywide average. Other well-known examples include Johns Hopkins Hospital, located in the Oldtown/Middle East neighborhood of Baltimore, which has a median annual household income of $14,105, a family poverty rate of 60 percent, and a lower life expectancy than the city's average.[19] The University of Chicago Medical Center sits in Hyde Park, where life expectancy is 82.7 years, while in the adjacent neighborhoods of Washington Park and Woodlawn, life expectancy drops to 70.4 and 75.3 years, respectively (Chicago's city average is 77).[20]

The presence of elite hospitals in neighborhoods with profound health and economic needs is not limited to a few isolated cases. Among the 100 top-ranked U.S. hospitals, nearly a quarter are in communities with diabetes and hypertension rates above the city averages and nearly half are in neighborhoods with higher-than-city-average asthma rates. Figure 1.1 provides specific examples of places where health outcomes in areas surrounding top-ranked medical centers differ the most (positively or negatively) from the city as a whole.

Proximity to a major hospital, in other words, is at times associated with *worse* health outcomes.[21] This does not mean that large hospitals are the primary or direct cause of poor health in surrounding communities, but it does suggest that providing quality patient care does not guarantee that individuals residing nearby will have the same opportunities for good health. In response,

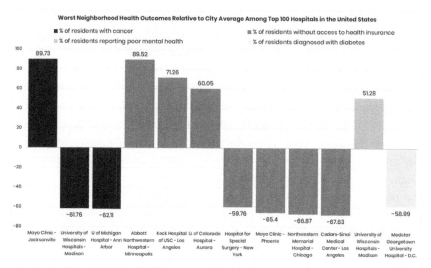

FIGURE 1.1. Top 12 most severe health outcomes relative to city average among top 100 U.S. hospitals
Source: Becker's Hospital Review: 100 Great American Hospitals in America; PLACES: Local Data for Better Health.

we ask: What are the missed connections, historical misunderstandings, and deliberate strategies that made this condition possible? Answering these questions requires interrogating the long-standing socioeconomic and racialized health disparities in the U.S. as well as understanding how policies and institutions have contributed to social inequality.[22]

While many hospitals can, and increasingly do, improve health not just for their individual patients but also in the neighborhoods and communities in which they are embedded, the causal question of *why* neighborhoods surrounding urban hospitals have comparatively poor health outcomes is complicated. Finding answers means looking past the glossy public relations material and well-crafted mission statements on hospital websites, and even beyond stellar clinical outcomes for hospital-based services. To understand the health of hospital-adjacent communities, this chapter sets the stage for the remaining text by providing an abridged history of American healthcare, presenting local profiles of our hospitals and the city neighborhoods they inhabit, and offering a robust picture of the healthcare conditions of the three cases.

A Brief Biography of Hospitals:
From Charity Care to Community Benefit

Prior to the nineteenth century, hospitals mainly focused on providing charity care for the poor and vulnerable, serving as a place of refuge and rehabilitation, while wealthier and healthier persons received personalized care in their homes. Many people feared hospitals, and people of means paid to avoid them altogether.[23] Hospitals were often not spaces for recovery but rather sites visited out of necessity.

Responding to the long-held belief that "bad air" was a root cause of many ailments, founders built nineteenth-century hospitals as small buildings with fresh-air wards. These facilities improved upon the home-care model in terms of efficiency and cost and offered physicians the controlled conditions necessary for clinical practice and research. They were also somewhat removed from the communities they served. For example, in late 1800s Manhattan, eight of ten general hospitals were above 54th Street, an hour's horse ride from the population centers below 23rd Street.[24] Others, however, were in the heart of the city: Beth Israel and St. Vincent's were located nearer to dense residential populations, the former near the Jewish enclave of the Lower East Side and the latter on the West Side near an Irish Catholic immigrant population. Public funding meant general municipal hospitals had to admit all patients.[25]

U.S. hospitals proliferated in the early-to-mid-twentieth century, driven especially by the passage of the Hill-Burton Act of 1946, which authorized federal funding for hospital construction in underserved areas and "launched the nation on the most comprehensive hospital and public health construction program ever undertaken."[26] The Act, however, took a "separate but equal" approach, allowing hospitals to institutionalize racial discrimination within facilities.[27] As medicine advanced, hospitals increased their roles as hubs and training sites where members of the burgeoning medical profession gained legitimacy and prestige. The profession expanded its authority on matters related to health and well-being, and hospitals differentiated themselves from the mission of public health and a focus on social determinants of illness, preferring to focus on technological innovation and the development of the biomedical model of care, establishing medical expertise, and advancing individual-level patient care.[28]

The 1964 Civil Rights Act (as well as its subsequent orders and laws) required health facilities, including hospitals, to provide "meaningful access" to patients. Building on this important development was the landmark passage of Medicare and Medicaid in 1965, which gave the federal government additional leverage in local healthcare arrangements by attaching certain requirements (e.g., accessible emergency rooms, desegregated healthcare facilities) and changes to expectations for community engagement to federal funding. Although Medicaid remains the largest budget item in most states, the federal budget, which covers about two-thirds of total Medicaid expenditures, provides a wide range of benefits to healthcare institutions, especially reductions in uncompensated care delivered in emergency departments.

In 1986, Congress enacted a bill of great consequence to communities, leveraging Medicare funds to ensure that hospitals did not turn patients away without addressing their emergency medical needs to at least some extent. Encoded in Section 1867 of the Social Security Act, the Emergency Medical Treatment and Labor Act (EMTALA) "imposes specific obligations on Medicare-participating hospitals that offer emergency services to provide a medical screening examination when a request is made for examination or treatment for an emergency medical condition, including active labor, regardless of an individual's ability to pay."[29] Hospitals are required to provide care to such patients to the point of stabilization. While the direct aim and substantive effect of EMTALA was to afford legal protections to patients arriving in emergency departments, the bill set new expectations for hospitals to treat community members, including in situations where they may have previously erected barriers to access. As we will explain in chapter 4, EMTALA played a key role in converting emergency departments and their waiting rooms into "contact zones" with their neighborhoods. A great deal of discussion has been directed at these areas, with emergency departments serving as staging grounds for well-known healthcare phenomena such as patient dumping, surprise billing, and questions about immigration status in the provision of federally funded healthcare services.

Emergency departments have sat at the center of the larger story of healthcare for the better part of three decades. Yet the dismal economics of the U.S. healthcare system continues to exert pressure on hospitals in other ways as well. In the early 2000s, American hospitals felt increasing pressure and public outcry over aggressive debt collection practices and a lack of price transparency, including but not limited to emergency care.[30] The new narrative that key parts of the U.S. healthcare industry—from insurance and pharmaceutical companies to hospitals—were failing to meet basic expectations prompted President Barack Obama to prioritize healthcare reform in 2009 in the form of the ACA.

The ACA's focus was multifaceted, but the bill prioritized expanding healthcare access for the uninsured, improving the delivery of healthcare services, and financially supporting many public health activities. The expansion of Medicaid to new populations was a pivotal component of this healthcare law, not only reducing uncompensated care for hospitals, but also freeing up other resources, such as funding for interpretation services and support for access to healthful food.[31] The ACA also changed how nonprofit hospitals approach community benefit expectations because hospitals' previous practice of providing free and reduced-cost care in exchange for tax exemption would no longer be as consequential with many more Americans insured. Instead, the

ACA asked hospitals to address critical community health needs and expand their focus beyond patient care. In doing so, the ACA established a more rigorous set of reporting requirements for compliance than had been in place for much of the twentieth century.

Just prior to passage of the ACA, the Internal Revenue Service (IRS) introduced Schedule H, a supplement to Form 990, which hospitals file each year.[32] Among other things, Schedule H offered more specific language and guidance regarding the meaning of expenditures earmarked for community benefit. Two new concepts—"community health improvement" and "community building"—were also introduced. In 2020, the Government Accountability Office more clearly delineated what type of work constitutes community benefit while allowing that the nature of this work within the general categories should be flexible and not overly prescribed. This balance was intended to allow entities to attend to local circumstances and needs.[33] The IRS does require, however, that community benefit not be used explicitly for hospital marketing purposes or in ways that primarily benefit the hospital rather than the community.[34]

Even though changes in the IRS code and the passage of the ACA forced many hospitals to broaden their idea of community to include the communities at their back doors, and to offer a variety of services for the poor and uninsured in their surrounding neighborhoods, these changes sometimes led hospital personnel to describe the good work they see themselves as doing for this group as a compliance consideration related to federal community benefit requirements. For example, Heidi Gartland, Chief Government and Community Relations Officer at University Hospitals, noted: "Our charity actually went up from last year to this year, and our total community benefit went up significantly. And again, we don't budget for it. We just do what we think the community needs, and I feel really good that we're making investments." Similarly, Greg Jones, Vice President for Community Health and Engagement at Hartford HealthCare, noted that the entire Hartford HealthCare system spends "roughly $280 million in community benefit. About half of that, maybe more, 60 percent of that—$175 million roughly—is unreimbursed financial care."

Although the ACA formally requires public hospitals to provide services to the broader public, the segregation shaping the communities outside hospitals also shaped the hospitals themselves. Many were founded on missions to care for targeted populations (e.g., Jews, Catholics, Presbyterians, or African Americans).[35] Accordingly, hospitals were often unequal in their care provision, with some differentiating patient care based on class, with charity wards for the poor, and others offering "separate but equal" treatment stratified by race.[36] Although passage of the Civil Rights Act of 1964, Medicaid, and

Medicare mandated desegregation in hospitals, clinical spaces and the neighborhoods around hospitals remained profoundly unequal.[37] In fact, many U.S. neighborhoods are almost as segregated as they were in the Jim Crow era, and acceptance of public insurance, such as Medicaid, still varies depending on the racial composition of local communities.[38] While a patient from 1900 would be gobsmacked by the high-tech, antiseptic, and well-manicured citadels of care like Hartford's Bone and Joint complex, they would be less surprised by how difficult it is for neighborhood residents to access these clinical spaces.

Community benefit remains a central topic in conversations about what private nonprofit hospitals owe communities in return for their sizable tax exemptions. The idea of "community benefit" was first included in IRS code in the 1950s, but even before this time, nonprofit hospitals largely understood their obligations as centering on the provision of charity care for those who could not afford their services.[39] Language introduced in 1969 evolved and was strengthened under Revenue Ruling 69–545,[40] which was a step toward clarifying that community benefit transcended emergency department access and charity care; however, vague administrative rules and limited enforcement meant that these rules did not radically alter the community benefit landscape.

The ACA requires that private nonprofit hospitals conduct Community Health Needs Assessments (CHNAs) every three years, and our three hospitals have used these documents to identify important needs in their local neighborhoods. The resultant report must include an identification of concrete "implementation" strategies for addressing identified problems.[41] CHNAs sparked conversation among compliance and public health experts about what hospitals should be expected to do, and what the expectations for oversight would be. Yet the federal government has expressed little interest in aggressively pursuing hospitals that fail to make meaningful investments. Community benefit itself is often a vague notion, with the IRS itself noting that "no one factor is determinative in considering whether a nonprofit hospital meets the community benefit standard."[42] These national policies and developments—as well as others discussed later in the book—shaped the trajectories of the three case communities; however, local histories influenced these healthcare landscapes just as significantly.[43]

Three Cases: History and Health

The areas we studied were typical of many urban neighborhoods surrounding hospitals. While we present detailed data throughout the book, suffice it to say that the neighborhoods we examined are largely communities of color and some of the poorest districts in their cities, with low homeownership rates, frequent evictions, high mobility and transience, and low rates of owner-occupied dwellings. All are experiencing the familiar results of historical red-lining and decades of disinvestment and white flight.[44] At the same time, the hospitals we focused upon have their own histories, occasionally intersecting with neighborhood histories (see fig. 1.2).

UNIVERSITY OF COLORADO HOSPITAL, ANSCHUTZ MEDICAL CAMPUS, AURORA, COLORADO

Currently the 19th largest city in the U.S., Denver, Colorado, is growing fast; its population expanded by over 20 percent between 2010 and 2020. Its neighbor to the east, Aurora, where the University of Colorado Hospital is currently located, is also growing rapidly, not only in population but also in investment and—as most residents will say—promise. In many ways, Aurora sits in the shadow of Denver, searching for its own identity.[45] Denverites tend to regard Aurora as a suburb.[46] Whereas Denver is a bustling city with a downtown skyline nestled in the Rockies, Aurora is attracting new capital to its growing downtown, and is home to a continuous flow of domestic and international immigrants that make it one of the country's most diverse cities.[47]

For decades, Aurora was a military town, starting with the establishment of Army General Hospital #21 in 1918 and culminating in a chain of Air Force and Air National Guard bases in eastern Denver and western Aurora. While Buckley Airforce Base in eastern Aurora is still the largest employer, the city was not immune to the post-war military base realignment and closures of the 1990s. The 1995 announcement of the closing of the Fitzsimons Army Medical Center sparked a reshuffling of Denver's medical institutions.[48] The center of the Anschutz Medical Campus still houses an impressive building that links the healthcare center to its military past. "Building 500" (the old Fitzsimons Hospital, renamed Fitzsimons in 2018), an art deco architectural gem, in 1955 housed President Eisenhower after he experienced a heart attack while golfing.[49] During an interview with the Vice President for Government and Corporate Relations, we toured Eisenhower's room as well as a large building that contains the mail facilities for the booming Anschutz Medical Campus and a rooftop observatory where large medical facilities were being erected as part of the continuing transformation from military base to regional medical center.

The University of Colorado Hospital was built on the main University of Colorado campus in Boulder, Colorado, but soon after moved 30 miles to downtown Denver, where it remained for the next 83 years. After reaching the limits of expansion and facing resistance from its affluent and well-organized

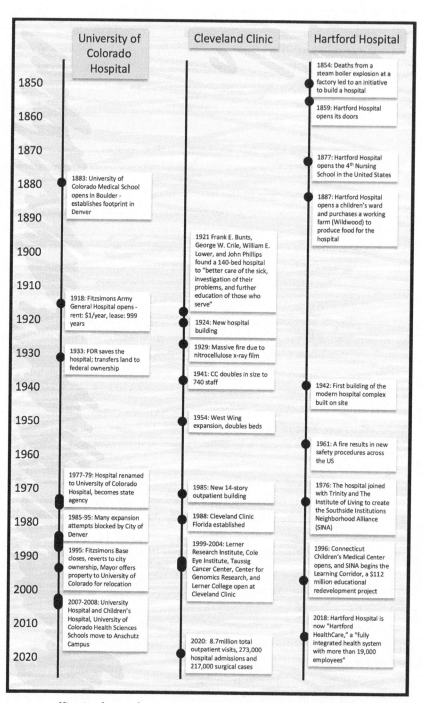

	University of Colorado Hospital	Cleveland Clinic	Hartford Hospital
1850			1854: Deaths from a steam boiler explosion at a factory led to an initiative to build a hospital
1860			1859: Hartford Hospital opens its doors
1870			
			1877: Hartford Hospital opens the 4th Nursing School in the United States
1880	1883: University of Colorado Medical School opens in Boulder - establishes footprint in Denver		1887: Hartford Hospital opens a children's ward and purchases a working farm (Wildwood) to produce food for the hospital
1890			
1900		1921 Frank E. Bunts, George W. Crile, William E. Lower, and John Phillips found a 140-bed hospital to "better care of the sick, investigation of their problems, and further education of those who serve"	
1910			
1920	1918: Fitzsimons Army General Hospital opens - rent: $1/year, lease: 999 years	1924: New hospital building	
1930	1933: FDR saves the hospital; transfers land to federal ownership	1929: Massive fire due to nitrocellulose x-ray film	
1940		1941: CC doubles in size to 740 staff	1942: First building of the modern hospital complex built on site
1950		1954: West Wing expansion, doubles beds	
1960			1961: A fire results in new safety procedures across the US
1970	1977-79: Hospital renamed to University of Colorado Hospital, becomes state agency	1985: New 14-story outpatient building	1976: The hospital joined with Trinity and The Institute of Living to create the Southside Institutions Neighborhood Alliance (SINA)
1980	1985-95: Many expansion attempts blocked by City of Denver	1988: Cleveland Clinic Florida established	
1990	1995: Fitzsimons Base closes, reverts to city ownership, Mayor offers property to University of Colorado for relocation	1999-2004: Lerner Research Institute, Cole Eye Institute, Taussig Cancer Center, Center for Genomics Research, and Lerner College open at Cleveland Clinic	1996: Connecticut Children's Medical Center opens, and SINA begins the Learning Corridor, a $112 million educational redevelopment project
2000			
2010	2007-2008: University Hospital and Children's Hospital, University of Colorado Health Sciences Schools move to Anschutz Campus		2018: Hartford Hospital is now "Hartford HealthCare," a "fully integrated health system with more than 19,000 employees"
2020		2020: 8.7million total outpatient visits, 273,000 hospital admissions and 217,000 surgical cases	

FIGURE 1.2. Histories of case studies

Sources: Cleveland Clinic, n.d., https://onbrand.clevelandclinic.org/learn-our-story/our-history/; Clouette and Lever 2004, https://www.cuanschutz.edu/about.

neighbors, the University of Colorado and the City of Aurora initiated conversations about the Fitzsimons site, which had closed by the end of June 1999. The old base was sold for a symbolic sum of $1.00, and the construction of the large multi-facility academic health center in Aurora began immediately (see fig. 1.3).

The story of what would eventually become the Anschutz Medical Center—named after Colorado billionaire business executive and philanthropist Philip Anschutz, who bankrolled much of its construction—is a tale of urban development as much as of healthcare. While downtown Denver's more affluent communities opposed expansion, the long-struggling city of Aurora was attracted to the promise of a new medical center. The diverse community of North Aurora, like many Colorado areas, experienced a tightening of the housing market over the past decade or so, displacing many residents. The expansion of healthcare facilities, in fact, might have been even more dramatic if not for the 2008 economic downturn that corresponded with the campus's opening. The nexus of medical institutions and emerging medical technology corporations was attractive to many developers, who purchased real estate in the surrounding neighborhoods only to flounder and eventually fold in the years after the recession.

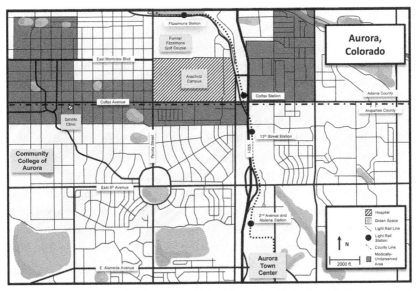

FIGURE 1.3. University of Colorado Anschutz Medical Campus and its Medically Underserved Areas/Populations (MUA/P)
Sources: Map designed by Wynn, based on OpenStreetMaps © OpenStreetMap contributors and MUA/P Data from HRSA (2022 Data).

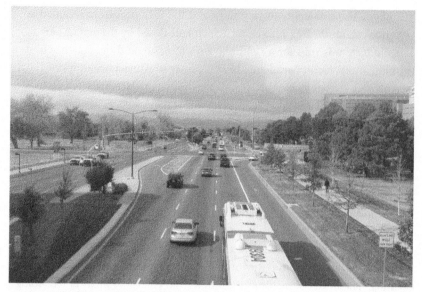

FIGURE 1.4. Looking west from the Colfax overpass connecting Anschutz's main facilities on the north and administrative buildings, as well as hotels and restaurants. University of Colorado Hospital is on the right. (Photo by Skinner)

Mirroring national trends, Aurora experienced several years of economic stagnation beginning in 2008 followed by a dramatic increase in development. In addition to welcoming the new medical community, Aurora was home to new developments in hospitality, aerospace, and defense as well as a half-million-square-foot Amazon processing facility and infrastructure projects, such as the light rail line connecting the city to Denver and Denver International Airport, all of which contributed to the city's growth.[50] Though Anschutz was in the unique position of being able to take over an abandoned military facility, which served as the foundation of its sprawling new campus, other hospital relocations or expansions capitalize on large-scale blight, including buying up abandoned or foreclosed homes.

As a result of the development, Aurora became the location of several of the region's preeminent university-affiliated medical institutions, educational facilities and, most recently (in 2018), the Rocky Mountain Regional VA Medical Center. With the exception of a few administrative buildings, the Anschutz Medical Center sits along Colfax Avenue, a 26.1-mile, largely pedestrian-unfriendly six-lane thoroughfare that also serves as the border between Adams and Arapahoe counties (see fig. 1.4).

Despite this growth, Aurora—especially the areas abutting the medical center—continues to report lagging economic and health indicators. The Anschutz Medical Campus is in a census tract designated by the U.S. Department of Housing and Urban Development (HUD) as a "qualified census tract," meaning it has high rates of poverty and is a difficult development area where land prices are out of line with the median income (see fig. 1.5, below). Uninsurance rates are one measure of access to medical services (nationally, 8.6 percent of Americans did not have health insurance at some point during 2020)[51]—while Aurora's average uninsurance rate is 15.8 percent, the neighborhoods abutting or near the campus report uninsurance rates ranging from 22 percent to 25 percent.

CLEVELAND CLINIC, CLEVELAND, OHIO

While Aurora is a diverse and sprawling mid-tier American city experiencing a population and development boom, the onetime fifth largest U.S. city of Cleveland, Ohio, has experienced a precipitous and steady loss of industry and population since the 1950s. Yet downtown Cleveland—if not the entire city—has also seen something of a renaissance in recent years as city stakeholders court new residents and businesses.

Three surgeons and an internist founded the Cleveland Clinic in 1921, locating the first buildings on Cleveland's historic East Side district, abutting the Fairfax and Hough neighborhoods. Expansion came quickly. By 1924, the trio had built a 184-bed hospital that included operating rooms, medical resident housing, and laboratories that were eventually folded into a dedicated research building. According to founder William Lower, "trading in land became an interesting game of chess for the Clinic and the property owners on East 93rd Street between Euclid and Carnegie."[52] In 1929, a fire from ignited nitrocellulose X-ray films killed 123 people and damaged much of the nascent campus; the newly rebuilt facility transformed the Clinic into a major medical center.[53]

Sitting at the north end of Euclid Avenue, on a four-mile strip once called "Millionaires' Row" due to its parade of Gilded Age mansions, the Hough and Fairfax neighborhoods experienced an influx of African American residents during the Great Migration out of the U.S. South, as Cleveland's population grew 60 percent between 1910 and 1930.[54] In the 1960s, as white residents fled to the suburbs, the neighborhood became a hub for Black culture and was home to several Black-owned businesses. In 1968, the Hough Riots erupted—three days of looting and violence in response to persistent local and national racial discrimination.[55] At the time, the Clinic's Board of Governors debated moving the hospital to the eastern suburbs but decided to not only stay, but expand. Soon after, the Clinic began a campaign of purchasing land, demolishing the existing buildings, and erecting new ones.

The 1990s saw a fresh wave of expansion, bolstered by the Clinic's increased emphasis on inpatient hospital services.[56] With increased affiliations and mergers of various regional hospital systems across the country,[57] the Clinic integrated multiple hospitals in the Cleveland area, creating the Cleveland Clinic Health System and prompting a hiring spree that propelled the Clinic into the city's top five employers. Throughout the late 1990s and early 2000s, the Clinic opened a series of primary care centers across the city and 10 additional campuses in Ohio as well as sites in Florida, Nevada, Toronto, Abu Dhabi, and London.[58] The Clinic's main campus is ranked second nationally overall and operates as a specialty hospital with patients coming from around the world.

In 2005, the Cleveland Foundation brought together the area's anchor institutions—the Cleveland Clinic, University Hospitals, Case Western Reserve University, the Cleveland Museum of Art, and the Cleveland Orchestra—to form the Greater University Circle Initiative (GUCI). This public-private collaboration is a bounded medical, cultural, and education district with the stated aim of "rebuild[ing] neighborhoods and improv[ing] the economic opportunities of the people who live" therein.[59]

Despite the growth and impressive rankings of the Clinic, and the collective efficacy of the GUCI institutions, the areas around University Circle lag in basic health indicators relative to the wider city.[60] Hough (to the west) and Fairfax (to the south of Euclid) host some of the highest morbidity rates in the city and nation. Infant mortality rates are three times the national average.[61] Cleveland's overall uninsurance average is 16.5 percent, but 19 percent of the population is uninsured in the Fairfax neighborhood. Diabetes rates also reveal stark disparities; the rate in the city is 16 percent, it nearly doubles to 31 percent in Fairfax, and then plummets to 7 percent in the affluent University Circle neighborhood to the east.[62] A local healthcare reporter we interviewed summarized these disparities, explaining, "Public health issues like lead poisoning, like infant mortality, pretty much any [issue] that you could possibly name. They all disproportionately affect the same neighborhoods in the city." By identifying Medically Underserved Areas, a map of the city is painted in stark condition (see fig. 1.5).

Another Clevelander, Jenny, who works at a local university, noted that the vulnerability of residents living near the Clinic was exacerbated by the Great Recession. She commented, "Some of the hardest-hit neighborhoods in the state are right next to these campuses. [Hospital employees] were seeing

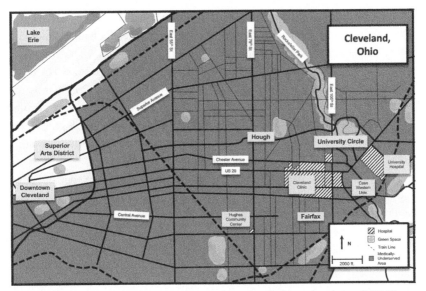

FIGURE 1.5. Cleveland Clinic Campus and its Medically Underserved Areas/Populations (MUA/P)
Sources: Map designed by Wynn, based on OpenStreetMaps © OpenStreetMap contributors and MUA/P
HRSA Data (2022).

it firsthand as they drove right past them on their way into the office every day." Respondents in Aurora and Hartford made similar comments about the Great Recession.

In addition, infant mortality rates on Cleveland's East Side (over 20 per 1,000 live births) are more than double the Cuyahoga County average (7.65 per 1,000 live births) and the U.S. average (6 per 1,000 live births).[63] There is consensus that racial disparities are driving these poor health outcomes, just as they do in urban communities across the U.S. Black women, for example, are three times more likely than white women to experience the loss of a child before their first birthday. Racial disparities hold even when controlling for important determinants of health (e.g., education level, income, and access to healthcare).[64] These statistics reveal a startling pattern: the infant mortality rate just outside the doors of a renowned medical institution is higher than the rates in many countries classified as "developing."[65]

HARTFORD HOSPITAL, HARTFORD, CONNECTICUT

Like Cleveland, Hartford was once a large and thriving American city. A one-time manufacturing hub known for producing firearms, hardware, and bicycles, Hartford now hosts only a third of the manufacturing jobs it had only a few decades ago. White-collar jobs tell an even bleaker story: Hartford was once the insurance capital of the country, earning it the nickname "America's Filing Cabinet," but major insurance companies (e.g., Aetna, The Hartford, and Travelers) partially or wholly fled to the suburbs or out of state. The city's population trajectory mirrors the patterns in many other New England and Northeastern cities, namely, a peak in the 1950s followed by a steady decline due to intense deindustrialization, suburbanization, and white flight. Hartford, which is the country's 227th largest city, is now one of the poorest cities in the country, with one in three residents living in poverty.

The capital of the nation's wealthiest state has teetered on the edge of bankruptcy for years. The remaining insurance companies provide only 20 percent of the tax base and, in 2017, a group of them agreed to donate $10 million per year for the next five years to prevent the city's bankruptcy.[66] Hartford's largest institutions—the government, hospitals, and institutions of higher education—comprise 51 percent of the properties in the city, all non-taxable. As in other cities, these "Eds and Meds" have been resistant to "Payment in Lieu of Taxes" (PILOTs) like those private-sector firms offered the city. Half a mile south of Hartford City Hall sits one of these tax-exempt property owners: Hartford Hospital.

Hartford Hospital's history begins on a pivotal day: March 2, 1852. At Dutch Point, a neighborhood only a few blocks from the hospital's present location, a steam boiler at a railroad car factory exploded, killing 19 and seriously injuring 23. In the aftermath of the disaster, the city's Protestant merchants and manufacturers, the Hartford Medical Society, and the *Hartford Courant* pushed for legislation to create a hospital. Founded in 1854 on the principles of charity and Christian duty, Hartford Hospital primarily treated immigrants and the working poor, as wealthy patients could afford to be treated at home.

As the only New England institution outside Boston that offered post–medical school training, Hartford Hospital grew quickly. Its exclusion of Jewish and Catholic interns from training prompted the city's Catholic population to open St. Francis Hospital in 1899 and the Jewish community to found Mount Sinai Hospital in 1923. St. Francis and Mount Sinai merged in 1995.[67]

As in other cities, infrastructure shaped Hartford's fortunes. The construction of the Interstate-84 viaduct, completed in 1965, created dead spaces and blight in the areas around Hartford Hospital, facilitated suburbanization and white and capital flight (as one commentator put it: those who work in Hartford's downtown do not commute so much as they "escape"[68]), and effectively bisected the city, demarcating the hospital regions: Mount Sinai and St. Francis to the north, Hartford Hospital to the south[69] (see fig. 1.6).

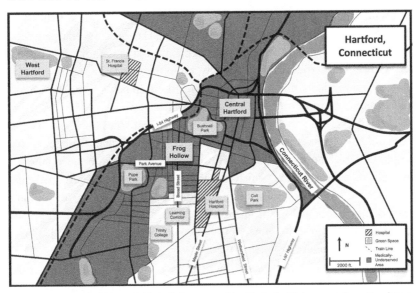

FIGURE 1.6. Hartford Hospital Medical Campus and its Medically Underserved Areas/Populations (MUA/P)

Sources: Map designed by Wynn, based on OpenStreetMaps © OpenStreetMap contributors and MUA/P HRSA Data (2022).

Three major steps (the first two mentioned at the top of the chapter) expanded the reach of Hartford Hospital in the last several decades. First, in 1994, the hospital acquired the Institute of Living, a behavioral health center with over 3,000 inpatients, set amid 35 acres of Frederick Law Olmsted–designed landscape across the street from the hospital. Second, the new Bone and Joint Institute opened in 2016. Third, in line with national trends toward healthcare consortiums, Hartford Hospital expanded into a hospital system—Hartford HealthCare—that owns and partners with six other acute care hospitals across the state as well as three behavioral health facilities and has established clinics to compete with hospitals in the suburbs.

The most populous of the communities surrounding the hospital is Frog Hollow—a name that refers to either the swamp that was once nearby or the French population that once lived there.[70] Interstate-84, the hospital, and Trinity College border the now predominantly Hispanic neighborhood.

The Southside Institutions Neighborhood Alliance (SINA) is a community organization that serves as a conduit between Frog Hollow and other adjacent communities and their anchor institutions, similar to the Greater University Circle Initiative but with a much smaller administrative budget and staff. SINA is funded primarily by Hartford Hospital, Connecticut Children's Medical Center (which sits adjacent to the Hartford Hospital campus), and Trinity College. The organization's explicit mission is similar to GUCI's: to stabilize the surrounding community, build better relationships with employees and residents, and help shape the relationship between neighborhood and community, most notably the Learning Corridor.

As in Cleveland and Aurora, the communities adjacent to or just beyond Hartford Hospital's campus have comparatively poor health outcomes. For example, the U.S. Census has designated the hospital's neighborhood as a health professional shortage area,[71] which means that, in addition to being "medically underserved" more generally, the neighborhood has a shortage of primary care, dental, or mental health providers. Further, while Hartford's uninsurance rate is 12.5 percent (compared to 19 percent nationwide),[72] Frog Hollow's rate is approximately 25 percent. Like Aurora and Cleveland, Hartford has a diabetes rate (14 percent) exceeding the national rate of 9 percent, while in Frog Hollow this rate jumps to 17 percent. In addition, the zip codes that encompass Frog Hollow, 06106 and 06114, are some of the state's poorest, with a homeownership rate of less than 10 percent and other key indicators worse than Hartford and state averages.

Circles of Disparity: Moving from Hospitals into Communities

To identify the current health patterns created by the local histories in these three communities, we examined health outcomes in several dimensions in the areas immediately around our three hospitals. Table 1.1 shows that the tracts contiguous to hospital land tend to rate poorly on five key variables assessing housing conditions (e.g., a large number of census tracts with high vacancy rates) but diverge on other indicators (e.g., over 60 percent of the population reported having a physical checkup in the previous year in all census tracts surrounding the Cleveland Clinic and Hartford Hospital, but in only a fraction of the tracts surrounding the University of Colorado).

Figure 1.7 shows that census tracts bordering our three hospitals have a higher likelihood of being designated a Medically Underserved Area and a "difficult to develop" area than the neighborhoods that are one, and especially two, census tracts away. Table 1.2 shows how the neighborhoods around the three hospitals fare on 12 health metrics compared with city and national averages: Aurora and Cleveland's immediate surrounding neighborhoods have health outcomes worse than national and city averages, while the neighborhood surrounding Hartford Hospital fares slightly better than the rest of the city on the same measures. And then table 1.3 provides a comparison of these

TABLE 1.1. Percentage of census tracts contiguous to hospital on five social, economic, and health variables

	Aurora (8 tracts)	Cleveland (9 tracts)	Hartford (8 tracts)
Low income/low food access @ 1–10 miles	37%	0%	0%
>15% of all business addresses vacant	12.5%	22%	12.5%
>10% of all residential addresses vacant	100%	78%	87.5%
>60% reporting physical checkup in last year	12.5%	100%	100%
>15% without healthcare insurance coverage	87.5%	44%	25%

Source: Social and economic factors and demographic data come from the U.S. Census Bureau. All other data come from the 500 Cities Project, which provides data on 500 city averages.

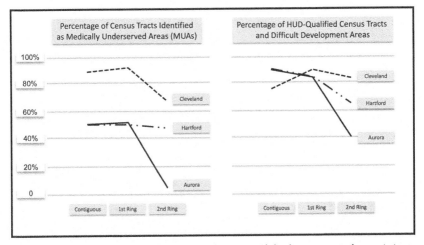

FIGURE 1.7. Neighborhoods' Medically Underserved Area and development status by proximity to hospitals
Source: U.S. Census Bureau and American Community Survey.
Note: Census tracts contiguous with hospital boundaries, compared with the next two "rings" of tracts. "Low-Income Housing Tax Credit Qualified Census Tracts must have 50 percent of households with incomes below 60 percent of the Area Median Gross Income (AMGI) or have a poverty rate of 25 percent or more. Difficult Development Areas (DDA) are areas with high land, construction and utility costs relative to the area median income and are based on Fair Market Rents, income limits, the 2010 census counts, and 5-year American Community Survey (ACS) data" (Office of Policy Development and Research, n.d.).

hospital neighborhood demographics as compared with the rest of their cities: overall, residents in these communities tend to be less white, more impoverished, more likely to be unemployed, and less likely to have health insurance.

Although COVID-19 data remains limited at the census tract level, we know from recent research that these health and economic disparities were strong predictors of severe COVID-19 illness and mortality and are inversely related

TABLE 1.2. Relative prevalence of health outcomes in hospital neighborhoods relative to city averages (shading indicates neighborhood prevalence is greater than the city average; bolded text indicates neighborhood prevalence is greater than the national average)

	Aurora	Cleveland	Hartford
High blood pressure	+6%	+15%	−8%
Cancer	−11%	+7%	−9%
Asthma	+7%	+6%	−6%
Heart disease	+21%	+21%	0%
COPD	+17%	+9%	−4%
Smoking	+22%	−3%	−2%
Diabetes	+27%	+24%	−4%
High cholesterol	+6%	+2%	−.2%
Chronic kidney disease	+19%	+24%	0%
Poor mental health	+18%	+1%	+1%
Obesity	+21%	+5%	−4%
Stroke	+26%	+36%	−8%

TABLE 1.3. Hospital neighborhoods compared with overall city demographics

	Unemployment	No health insurance	Poverty	White	Black/African American	Hispanic/Latino
Aurora	+203%	+124%	+150%	−63%	+1%	+80%
Cleveland	+204%	+32%	+53%	−44%	+38%	−84%
Hartford	+220%	+20%	+44%	−39%	−52%	+25%

Source: U.S. Census Bureau.

Note: Census tracts contiguous with hospital boundaries as compared with city census tract data.

to vaccination rates in U.S. communities. Indeed, studies have shown that factors such as social vulnerability and residential segregation are essential to understanding racial/ethnic, socioeconomic, and geographic disparities in COVID-19.[73] These data suggest that urban hospitals serve communities that are not only disproportionately at risk for chronic disease and economic distress, but also public health epidemics both presently and in the future. Additional health outcome data and social and demographic data for all three cases and city and national averages are available in Appendix B.

What does this view of the periphery mean for the hospitals that sit at the center? Given the variation in health indicators in these three communities, it is perhaps unsurprising that there is tremendous variation in community benefit spending across these institutions, especially relative to the nonprofit hospitals' operating expenses. Tax-exempt private hospitals such as Hartford Hospital and the Cleveland Clinic are required to report their community benefit spending, while the University of Colorado Hospital, which is a state agency, does not have the same requirements, though University of Colorado documents, as well as our interviewees, make clear that the institution regards itself as fully engaged in the same basic activities (e.g., CHNAs, community building programming) as private nonprofits. Figure 1.8 shows community benefit spending at the main campuses of Hartford Hospital and the Cleveland Clinic.[74] Appendix C provides examples of needs identified by all three hospitals/campuses as well as programs proposed or developed to address those needs as part of IRS-mandated implementation strategies.

In 2022, the Lown Institute Hospital Index determined that 82.5 percent of private nonprofit hospitals had a "fair-share deficit," meaning they spent less on charity care and community investment than they received in tax breaks. This was an increase from 72 percent in 2021. According to the index, the deficit totaled $18.4 billion; amounts varied widely across individual hospitals, from a few thousand dollars to hundreds of millions of dollars.[75] This assessment provides a rough guide for how these hospitals use their resources (see table 1.4). While the American Hospital Association disputes this assessment,[76] there remains a lack of clarity regarding key metrics for understanding how community benefit requirements help reduce health disparities and might improve overall outcomes in neighborhoods near hospitals and medical centers.

Municipal, state, and even national economic trends provide a more nuanced context for understanding community benefit. In many cases, hospitals could certainly do more.[77] Yet austerity budgeting, the defunding of social services and supports, and the erosion of local tax bases have an acute impact

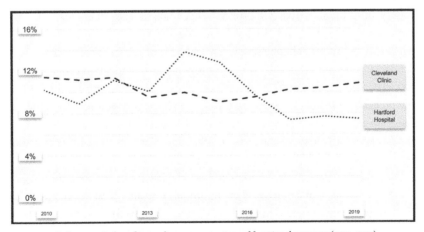

FIGURE 1.8. Community benefit spending as a percentage of functional expenses (2010–2019)
Source: IRS Form 990, Schedule H, retrieved from www.communitybenefitinsight.org.

TABLE 1.4. 2022 Community benefit report card

	University of Colorado Hospital (ranking in Colorado)	Cleveland Clinic (ranking in Ohio)	Hartford Hospital (ranking in Connecticut)
Overall social responsibility ("Reflects performance across health equity, value, and outcomes")	A (9th of 62)	A (26th of 130)	B (15th of 26)
Equity ("Reflects commitment to inclusivity, pay equity, and community investment")	B (27th of 66)	C (108th of 136)	C (19th of 26)
Community benefit ("Reflects how well hospitals invest in community health")	B (23rd of 64)	D (132nd of 135)	B (17th of 26)
Inclusivity ("Reflects how well hospitals serve people of color, people with lower incomes, and people with lower levels of education")	B (12th of 59)	B (83th of 132)	C (17th of 26)
Value ("Reflects how efficiently hospitals deliver care and avoid low-value services")	A (2nd of 62)	A (3rd of 130)	A (10th of 26)

Source: Lown Institute (https://lownhospitalsindex.org). For details on Lown's methodology, see https://lownhospitalsindex.org/rankings/our-methodology/.

on all three sites.[78] In Hartford, for example, Mary Stuart, Director of Health Equity at St. Francis Hospital, pointed to changes in the public health infrastructure on the state and city level. Stuart explained, "Part of the issue and part of what you see is happening is that public health is being completely unfunded at the state and local level. [Funding] needs to happen in order for this model to shift. If you don't have any resources at the state and local level for public health the hospital ends up trying to create those resources."[79] During these times of budgetary stress, the stable presence of an anchor institution such as Hartford Hospital can stand in stark contrast to the tumult of city and state budgeting.

Clearly, there are deeply entrenched health disparities in these communities despite persistent discussions about how community benefit expenditures and programming might address these disparities. Importantly, there is often a mismatch between what residents, hospital administrators, and other actors expect from these hospitals. While chapter 5 explores the question of expectations in detail, it is worth summarizing here. When talking about the Cleveland Clinic, Mansfield Frazier, for example, said bluntly that its "business is medicine," not community health. "The proof is," he continued, "Hough has an infant mortality rate higher than [those] in third-world countries, yet we're sitting right at the front door of one of the richest medical institutions in the world. How is that?" Another local leader, Kurt, had a more sympathetic perspective: "Their core business is treating the sick of our community and in helping people heal or stay well; they're so good at it. And that—I don't think that should be underestimated, 'cuz that's not easy, right? That's heroic." Overall, residents we spoke with either expected very little from these otherwise venerable institutions or were understandably perplexed as to why their medical institutions can develop groundbreaking innovations inside their walls but cannot find a way to stimulate meaningful change in the surrounding communities.

In Aurora, two hospital administrators discussed the implications of transitioning from an affluent neighborhood in Denver to Aurora. Dwight explained that the change in the health profile of the surrounding community motivated a change in perspective: "We literally moved from a prime neighborhood to a . . . neighborhood that hadn't even started [to] transition yet, so there was a clear need for us to play a bigger role as a better neighbor because it was a problem, the neighborhood was a problem." Dwight's colleague, Joe, described the move as an opportunity for new community engagement. He saw the City of Aurora "roll out the red carpet for us," but also recognized the pressure from the community. He characterized the community's perspective as wondering, "So, other than providing that healthcare, what else are you going to do for us?" Sometimes, in other words, local demands compel hospitals to become involved in community-focused work.

In Cleveland and Hartford, hospital and local leaders believe the emphasis should be on promoting the hospital's clinical, research, and teaching mission, rather than improving access. Some of these leaders see the provision of any services as a real benefit to the larger region, even if residents of nearby neighborhoods do not benefit directly. Michael, a physician at the Cleveland Clinic, argued the institution shouldn't lose focus on its mission of providing specialty care at the main campus. He contended the Clinic is "literally not intended or constructed to be a community resource." He described the work of physicians at the Clinic as doing "really complex things," including deep brain stimulation and heart transplants. And yet, he noted that the Clinic has had to envision itself as a community resource "by necessity because people will show up at your door whether you like it or not."

What, then, is the hospital's mission? Where do its primary responsibilities lie—with the medical research and care inside, or with the city that lies out-side its walls? While institutional mission statements are a particularly plati-tudinous genre, and possibly more public relations than actual practice, they can be seen as formal attempts by institutions to shape perceptions, both in-side the organization and externally in their various communities.

A hospital's sense of purpose can shape their approach to addressing health disparities and challenges. Kristen Morris of the Cleveland Clinic believed the hospital's role in addressing disparity is based on need, and the various pieces of the organization's mission fit together nicely: "The reason we are not-for-profit," Morris explained, "is that we do things the government would have to do if we didn't do it for them, such as manage public health and disease and poverty. We do a heck of a lot already." Morris noted the Clinic is the area's larg-est employer and even the largest taxpayer—when employee taxes are included. Beyond these considerations, Morris argued that "creating a healthier, more vibrant neighborhood" is the "emotionally [and] socially right thing to do."

In Hartford, a retired physician tried to thread the needle between the hos-pital's focus on clinical medicine and broader community needs. While ac-knowledging that the community had its own expectations, he said the hos-pital's "great commitment" to "educational capability, scholarly pursuits by the medical staff [and] even nonmedical staff" is a significant benefit to the community. In his view, the neighboring residents needed to appreciate that a teaching and research mission is a "community benefit," at least in the tech-nical sense of the term, though he recognized that neighbors might expect greater day-to-day impact. Residents, he continued, expect that whatever re-search the hospital does, it should connect directly with the public's needs. He paraphrased community sentiment as follows: "Do better telling us about our health. Tell us about our arthritis. Tell us about our heart trouble. Tell us about our dietary indiscretions that make us sick."

Hospital administrators generally accepted neighborhood health dispari-ties as multicausal facts that are only partially affected by the hospital's efforts to improve community health. A hospital administrator described the bal-ance of improving access to high-quality medical care and doing clinical work as both "saving lives and doing leading-edge clinical care [and] educating and training future health professionals and providing tremendous leading-edge research." Hospitals, however, rarely achieve this ideal balance. Just as resi-dents reflected on the paradox of health disparities, hospital administrators discussed how a greater awareness of population health reshapes their view of clinical care and how hospitals might influence community health. The ad-ministrators we interviewed agreed that their organizations should take this work seriously. As with residents, however, there was little consensus about what that means.

Despite differences of opinion regarding the best approach and the scope of this work, most hospital leaders agreed with residents that community-facing work must be part of hospitals' portfolios. Hartford Hospital's Greg Jones, in contrast, described a more individualistic model that largely excluded hospitals from the responsibility to respond to population health, emphasizing instead individuals' responsibility to attend to their own health. Jones asserted, "We all want to say it's the hospital's responsibility to build a community health center; it's the doctor's responsibility to help you. I say not." He noted this message was the central theme of the "Take Charge of Your Health" program he led at Hartford HealthCare.

Conclusion: Hospitals as Reluctant or Committed Anchors?

The health disparities and other challenges residents experience in the communities surrounding these hospitals shape the expectations of hospitals, neighborhood residents, and other stakeholders in key ways. Overall, most residents and hospital employees agreed that hospitals should focus on reducing health disparities in their surrounding neighborhoods. However, residents' views were more emphatic, universal, and focused on non-clinical care. Community members often simply wanted an expansion of access to quality healthcare, though, as noted in the introduction, there was often a palpable sense of caution about expressing these views publicly for fear of being denied future care.

The power these institutions hold within their respective communities is impressive and pervasive. As shown in the coming chapters, hospitals don't always appreciate the scope of their perceived power. At the same time, almost no one disputed the existence of race- and class-based health disparities in the urban neighborhoods surrounding each hospital. Participant opinions diverged, however, on the hospitals' responsibility for public health outcomes and the upstream social and economic factors shaping their community's health landscape. Chapter 2 explores the nature of hospital/community relationships, in both their historical and normative dimensions.

2

How History "Keys" the Hospital
and Community Relationship

> To this must be added a superstitious fear of hospitals prevalent among the lower
> classes of all people, but especially among Negroes. This must have some foundation
> in the roughness or brusqueness of manner prevalent in many hospitals, and the lack
> of a tender spirit of sympathy with the unfortunate patients. At any rate, many a Negro
> would almost rather die than trust himself to a hospital.
>
> W. E. B. DU BOIS, *The Philadelphia Negro*[1]

For a community, a singular story can epitomize the shortcomings of the U.S.
healthcare system. In our interviews, we encountered many such stories as well
as neighborhood memories that shaped and informed how respondents saw
their community's identity and history. While these narratives were context specific and often unique, they were also shaped by broader societal shifts (e.g.,
economic booms and busts, cultural changes in thinking about race). The narratives that determined people's shared meanings and values serve as what sociologists Hirschman and Reed call "formation stories."[2] In our contexts, specific stories shaped the community/hospital relationship, and they highlight
complicated histories around immigration status, race, and socioeconomic
status in these communities.

One such story concerned Eduardo Franco Ramirez. In September 2013,
muggers severely beat Ramirez, at that time an undocumented Guatemalan
immigrant and construction worker. Ramirez arrived at the University of Colorado Hospital's emergency department critically injured. Surgeons removed
a quarter of Ramirez's skull to reduce swelling around his brain and save his
life, and the hospital cared for him during a 16-day coma. When his condition
stabilized, however, the hospital explained that it was no longer required to
provide care under EMTALA.

Because the hospital is part of the University of Colorado Hospital Authority, a "political subdivision of the state" and not a private nonprofit hospital organization, hospital administrators decided not to provide further care
because Ramirez was not documented and did not have health insurance. To
justify their decision, they referenced a 2006 state law forbidding the use of
state funds to support charity care for undocumented residents. As a result, Ramirez was discharged with a helmet to protect the area where a piece of skull

had been removed.[3] The hospital argued that his condition was not an emergency and therefore they were not required to perform the surgery. After living in considerable pain for over a year, Ramirez had the surgery thanks to a crowdfunding campaign orchestrated by a local community organizer that raised $7,000.[4] Media coverage of the hospital's decision to discharge him with a piece of his skull missing also put tremendous pressure on the hospital to reverse course. The hospital agreed to do the procedure at one-tenth of the cost—the total amount of donations—in an effort to limit the embarrassment. Local coverage in *The Sentinel* emphasized the degree to which "community compassion" and not the efforts of local healthcare institutions was the key to Ramirez receiving care. The story quotes Rich McClean, the crowdfunding organizer to secure Ramirez's care, as offering an implicit criticism of the institutions. McClean explained, "That's probably going to be key in future Eduardo cases—the community has to be willing to step up and not be indifferent to that pain and suffering going on."[5] Although the hospital stepped up, it required community action and relationship development in the preceding years to get to that point.

McClean, who is a member of the Aurora Health Alliance, met us at a local coffee shop to discuss the efforts to secure Ramirez's surgery; he later drove us around the local neighborhood to explain the scope of collaborative work conducted over the last decade. As McClean explained, stories like the Ramirez saga show that hospitals sometimes fail to serve residents, but these failures can also serve as the baseline for more productive partnerships; further, these stories emphasize that improving health outcomes will require strengthening hospital/community relationships:

> At the lower levels, the doctors, the hands-on [staff], the providers—they truly care. They want to help. But they don't run the administration and they don't pay the bills. But they constantly are battling the hospital to open up doors of access to care. So that's kind of how we started working with the lower-level providers and helping them to make the case to the upper-level administrators of the hospital. [The Ramirez story] is an example of how this might not have happened 10 years ago or 8 years ago. But it happened now, basically because the community has a stronger relationship with the University than it had before. Again, there are many other folks out there that have dire conditions that don't have the publicity.

Residents in all three of our research sites clearly stated that the way hospitals engaged with the surrounding communities held a persistent and active place in the narratives of community members' collective memories. Some administrators also had an eye on history as an influential force. For example, David Crombie at Hartford Hospital explained:

As you trace the history of the relationship, you see times when the hospital said, "We are reliant upon the good graces of our prominent citizens to help us build a new building or buy a CAT scan," and on the other hand, when the community was down on its luck a little bit, during economic hard times, the community said, "You're a big institution. You're a large employer. We really need you to help us out too . . . rehabilitate neighborhoods, guide us in architectural maneuvers that might improve our city." You see over 150 years of this "I'm going to help you. I may need you tomorrow," and back and forth. The hospital was always a pretty stable partner with deep pockets, big endowment money, and [was] unafraid to make moves.

From Crombie's perspective, "the hospital stood up" when neighborhoods "became economically shaky." Yet he characterized the hospital/community relationship as interdependent, concluding, "The community says, 'We need a hospital.' The hospital says, 'We need the community.'"

Despite Crombie's description of interdependence, the nationwide hospital/community relationship is tenuous. A Denver-based professor described the influence of "formation stories" in the areas around the Anschutz campus: "Word travels fast . . . when you're expecting something and then it's not delivered . . . the narrative is, 'So-and-so showed up in an ambulance and they wouldn't take them and they sent them down to the next hospital . . .'" The professor noted that stories like these make a negative impression on residents, concluding, "People get a sense [that] this hospital really wasn't built for them."

Social and cultural factors can inform people's decision-making around health,[6] particularly for marginalized, excluded, or displaced residents. Understanding these community dynamics requires listening to patterns and repetitions and finding points of contention. On gaining access to local knowledge, Clifford Geertz noted that "to-know-a-city-is-to-know-its-streets,"[7] and research shows that local stories can point to the blind spots within organizations and urban institutions, particularly with communities at risk.[8] This chapter, then, explores how memories and histories have shaped the present relationships between hospitals and communities. Indeed, the health of the broader community can hinge on the content of these "formation stories."

Health and History in Communities of Color

These urban institutions, led primarily by white administrators, are not located in just any communities, but predominantly in communities of color. Many people we interviewed both inside and outside hospitals discussed this situation openly, taking part in a conversation even more vital within the wider political and cultural context of an increased national awareness of systemic racism.[9] Kenneth, a nonprofit worker in Cleveland, explained that part of his job when working with the Cleveland Clinic and other local entities is to ensure "that we keep structural and systemic racism at the table, at the conversation, because we do know that a lot of the current ails of the community is a direct result of structural racism."

Of course, the observation that hospitals are predominantly white institutions situated within communities of color is not a fresh insight.[10] Like most U.S. institutions and organizations, hospitals reproduce white privilege and power. In *How Racism Takes Place*, George Lipsitz explained the concept of a "white spatial imaginary" that can be applied to hospitals:

> [This imaginary] idealizes "pure" and homogeneous spaces, controlled environments, and predictable patterns of design and behavior. It seeks to hide social problems rather than solve them . . . This imaginary does not emerge simply or directly from the embodied identities of people who are white. It is inscribed in the physical contours or the places where we live, work, and play, and it is bolstered by financial rewards for whiteness.[11]

Recently, sociologists examining how shared collective trauma drives health disparities noted that *cultural* traumas differ from *interpersonal* traumas in that the former are assaults enacted by a dominant group when they damage, devalue, or destroy a group's key resources, and these effects are reinforced over time.[12]

These historical traumas can be nearly insurmountable obstacles in contemporary health and healthcare. A study of Canadian First Nations patients, for example, found that historical memory of how hospitals treated patients with tuberculosis decades prior undermined contemporary health utilization.[13] Similarly, decades of personal experiences, passed down across generations, shape how communities approach healthcare in the present.[14]

Some of the medical professionals we interviewed referenced this perspective. For example, Devorah, a resident who is also employed at Cleveland's MetroHealth hospital, recalled that when she told a hospital administrator she was encountering some hesitancy in the Black community, he asked her why African Americans don't avail themselves of free flu shots and vaccinations. She was stunned at his lack of awareness of the troubling and racist history of the medical field. "Don't y'all remember syphilis?" she asked him, referring to the Tuskegee Syphilis Study, the 40-year research project of withholding syphilis treatment in African American men supported by the U.S. Public Health Service. She continued educating the administrator, explaining, "It's just that simple. They don't trust you. They don't care what you give out for free."

Racism is deeply entrenched in the field of medicine. Kathy, a nonprofit leader in Cleveland, asserted that even though healthcare professionals know there are no "fundamental differences at a cellular level" across racial groups, they continue to engage in race-based medical practices, and patients of color continue to receive lower-quality care. Explicit segregation in medical settings is hardly a distant memory. In the nearby Glenville neighborhood, Forest City Hospital was founded by Black physicians in 1957 because the Cleveland Clinic did not admit white patients or employ Black healthcare professionals. Although Forest City transitioned away from acute inpatient care following the national desegregation of hospitals in the 1960s, racism persists in the quality of the care patients receive. Reminiscent of the enforced segregation of the past, current-day biological racism persists in the form of "race norming," or efforts to use race as a biological category when making treatment decisions for patients from different so-called racial groups. In practice, race norming includes using different pain thresholds for racial groups or applying different guidelines and corrections when interpreting patients' lab results.[15]

As shown in the well-known report *Unequal Treatment* (published by the Institute of Medicine, now the National Academy of Medicine), large, urban hospitals have treated and continue to treat patients differently based on race.[16] The reinvigorated commitment by many medical and public health institutions in the wake of persistent racial/ethnic health disparities and police brutality— itself a public health crisis—has led to explicitly medical movements including "White Coats for Black Lives." Major professional organizations, including the American Medical Association and the American Hospital Association, have issued calls for renewed efforts to address racial inequities in medicine.[17] Despite this growing recognition, however, the health gap between racial/ ethnic groups in the U.S. remains profound and is sometimes exacerbated by hospitals' clinical practices and their historical place in neighborhoods.[18]

We were surprised by moments when administrators spoke directly to how their institutions offered different treatment to patients and excluded neighborhood residents in the past. Many of our interviewees discussed efforts to address these histories and improve the conditions that serve as their legacies.

Almost without exception, hospital administrators believed change was afoot at higher levels of their institutions. Max, a local nonprofit leader in Cleveland, described the city as deeply segregated, and acknowledged that the hospital administration "couldn't avoid talking about it." He knew several staff and administrators who had read or were reading Michelle Alexander's *The New Jim Crow*. According to Max, the book's thesis—that the rise of mass incarceration in the U.S. was just the latest stage in legalized discrimination— left administrators "profoundly shocked and more committed to racial equity." Max told us that in addition to hospital staff reading about this topic, local programs such as Jump Start, Cleveland Neighborhood Progress, and the Racial Equity Institute provided racial awareness training to the hospital board and personnel. We heard of similar efforts in the other cities. For example, Max recalled an instance in which the Cleveland group met with a dean at the University of Colorado who acknowledged that hospitals needed to change their perspective from the historical view of their non-white poor neighboring communities as "a contagion to be suppressed" to a perception of these same residents as "an asset to be engaged with."

Yet for all this new awareness, few American medical institutions engage with their own histories in meaningful ways. There are a few notable exceptions: Georgetown University publicly recognized historical slaveholding and enacted a policy to provide legacy status and preferential admission to the descendants of individuals enslaved by the university.[19] Johns Hopkins University faced its past unauthorized use of cancer cells from Henrietta Lacks, a Black woman from the Baltimore area—a reckoning that included close consultation with Lacks's descendants in the development of plans to engage with local schools, put on symposia twice each year, and offer scholarships for high school students interested in pursuing science.[20] Administrators tend to speak with pride about this kind of historically engaged activity, but such work is rarely billed as a historical corrective. Locals may see the accomplishments for which many hospitals are applauded (e.g., important clinical discoveries and advances) as either irrelevant to their day-to-day concerns or as coming at the expense of providing care for the local communities.[21]

Deep Memories and Significant Community Moments

Reinaldo Rojas, a professor at Central Connecticut State University, studied community organizing in Hartford's Frog Hollow neighborhood for years. When asked about the history of the primarily Latin and Hispanic community and its relationship to the hospital, he recounted, with a great deal of enthusiasm mixed with anger, the story of how, in the 1970s, powerful players in city businesses and government secretly authored a plan to redevelop the downtown area—a plan that explicitly included displacing communities of color in the neighborhoods around Hartford Hospital. He noted that his conversations with residents revealed "a deep memory about these approaches."

The local histories in Aurora, Cleveland, and Hartford are embedded within these wider narratives, shaping the relationships communities have with their healthcare institutions. People may move in and out of these communities, but like the anchor institutions themselves, these stories are resilient, weaving themselves into the fabric of neighborhood memories.[22] Most recently, these deep memories have reemerged, fueling hesitancy about the administration of COVID-19 vaccines. This is, however, just the latest example among many.

The perspectives of both local residents and hospital employees offered insight into the contested terrain of a few common ideas—place, community, and trust. Being attuned to these themes provided us a clearer picture of the socially, culturally, and historically grounded barriers to healthcare that may persist even as healthcare broadens its focus to improve healthcare access by improving transportation, increasing health literacy, and addressing other documented barriers to healthcare utilization.

Rojas was not the only one to refer to a community's "deep memories." Interviewees in Aurora, Cleveland, and Hartford said that key historical events continue to shape contemporary relationships. Such significant moments, whether decades in the past or more recent, create crystalized shared sentiments in communities and mobilize individual dispositions and group actions. Sociologist Erving Goffman would have noted that these histories "key" sentiments and interactions.[23] Moreover, mistrust is not merely an objective consequence of histories, but rather a defense mechanism and can even serve as a strategic tool communities use to protect themselves. In each of the three cases, a longer view of hospital/community interactions is necessary to understand the current dynamics and the potential paths to success in any future population health efforts.

CLEVELAND: GROWTH IMPERATIVES MEET COMMUNITY RESISTANCE

Members of the local Black community put up resistance as the Cleveland Clinic rapidly expanded from a quaint "clinic" to a large urban campus with its own zip code. Fannie Lewis, the longest-serving city councilwoman in Cleveland history and one of the most prominent Black politicians in the city,[24] was reported to have successfully run her campaign in opposition to the hospital's growth, calling the Clinic "the devil" in her campaign speeches. Such fiery rhetoric galvanized some residents, likely contributing to her success in the nearby Hough neighborhood, but also made some local professionals uncomfortable. The problem, however, wasn't that these individuals disagreed with Lewis's criticism, but rather that they feared speaking against the Clinic could jeopardize future collaborations with an organization that had increasing influence over local city planning. These fears appear well founded given the experience of Winston Willis. Of all the stories interviewees told in East Cleveland, his loomed largest.

Willis, who died in November 2021, was a successful Black business owner and real estate developer. In the 1960s, he owned a number of businesses near 105th and Euclid Avenue, including a famous club called "The Jazz Temple," which hosted some of the most well-known musicians of the time—Miles Davis, John Coltrane, and Dizzy Gillespie all performed there.[25] As a powerful and well-known entrepreneur who employed over 400 other African Americans, Willis earned the nickname "the Black Rockefeller."

We spoke with Willis's sister, Aundra, who is dedicated to keeping his story alive and spreading the word about his confrontations with the Cleveland Clinic. She said that the 1966 and 1968 Hough and Glenville Riots—reactions to marginalization and poverty and accelerating white and capital flight in the area—not only heightened local tensions but also set the stage for the Clinic's expansion. The unrest devalued the properties in Hough, and the Clinic capitalized on this shift. Aundra explained that, as the Clinic began to buy up land in the area, Winston's properties were "in their way" and "he refused to leave."

Aundra believes this confrontation with the Clinic made Winston a target of the police, the city, the fire department, and the IRS. He spent millions in legal fees to challenge the legality of raids on his properties.[26] From her perspective, the city looked the other way while the Clinic, along with other developers, bought land near or adjacent to his properties and then left them vacant, leading to increased crime rates and lower property values. In response, Winston erected billboards to expose what he regarded as broad racism, corruption, and persistent injustice that African Americans experienced at the hands of both the city and the Clinic.[27] One of his signs, posted in 1982, read "Cleveland Clinic Strikes Again! Continues its elimination of blacks from this community. Food stores and Sears now gone. Big blow to blacks."

The harassment escalated. In 1988, police arrested Willis on a charge of writing bad checks and sent him to a prison 200 miles away. (His sister and others vehemently dispute the legality of the charges, saying he never signed the check in question.) While Willis sat in solitary confinement and was denied access to his lawyer, the city seized his assets and gifted his properties to the Cleveland Clinic. Later, Willis fought to regain his assets, taking his case all the way to the U.S. Supreme Court, where it was docketed and eventually denied with little explanation. Willis and his family members have never been compensated for their losses.[28]

When we interviewed Cleveland residents, they repeatedly mentioned Willis's name and story. Today, the W. O. Walker Rehabilitation Center, a Cleveland Clinic expansion project, stands on one of Willis's properties,[29] and there seems to be little chance for a return of the opportunity corridor Willis once

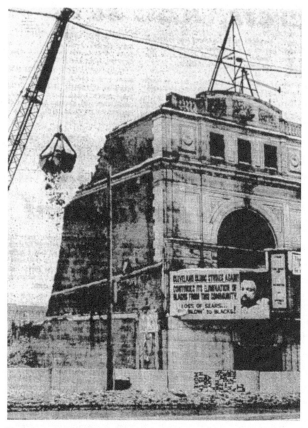

FIGURE 2.1. Newspaper clipping of Willis's last marquee message.
Source: *Cleveland Plain Dealer*, permissions granted.

built. A local professor, Max, described this history as a powerful demonstra-
tion of the ways racist policies contributed to land acquisition and shaped the
trajectory of the neighborhood, and said the story continues to stoke mistrust among residents. He explained, "It is something Black residents have
a deep memory [of] . . . Their view of the hospitals is not necessarily [that
they are] benevolent, and hospitals are aware of that." The racism and raw
institutional power exercised over the Black community was not surprising
to residents, nor were they shocked that a hospital would participate in this
type of violence.

For many Clevelanders, the Willis story is merely an exceptional example
of a pattern they had either experienced or observed. Courtney, a local community organizer, reported hearing similar stories. She recalled the Clinic's
purchase of a beautiful home on Euclid Avenue; while they received what the
family thought was a fair price, the Clinic razed the home and left the prop-

erty vacant. Both the family and the Black community perceived these actions as hurtful to neighborhood residents who have history there and were encouraged to sell as the Clinic developed the land nearby. Courtney told us how the family rides past the lot and, instead of feeling pride, they only see an empty lot. These types of stories, she remarked, show how the neighborhood has been "wiped out," undermining their shared sense of place.

Winston Willis's story intersects with broader histories of hospitals refusing to hire Black physicians and provide care to Black patients. Courtney, for example, linked the legacy of institutional discrimination to poor health outcomes in predominantly Black neighborhoods on Cleveland's East Side, where differences in life expectancy between Hough and nearby neighborhoods are as large as 20 years. Black residents in the communities around the Clinic, she observed, remember having to travel to Forest City Hospital, known as "Cleveland's interracial hospital" through the 1970s. Courtney concluded that the history of Hough "can't be ignored [because] it was racially driven during that time, and I mean, there's been some progress, but we are still living in racially charged times, and that impacts the health and wealth of communities." In conversations like these, memories of the hospital and the city treating the community poorly intersect with current opinions that the Clinic's successes come at the expense of communities of color such as Hough and Fairfax.

HARTFORD: WHICH COMMUNITY DOES A HOSPITAL ANCHOR?

Because the community surrounding Hartford Hospital has long been primarily Hispanic, Hartford's downtown has been a destination for new and undocumented immigrants for decades. The community is historically Puerto Rican, although new residents from Mexico, Colombia, Cuba, Peru, and other countries now gravitate to the area in part because a stable set of small businesses along the neighborhood's main commercial drag, Park Avenue, cater to these groups.

As in all cities, Hartfordites and local healthcare practitioners know fragments of the city's history. Sometimes these memories are worth celebrating, and sometimes they are not. Hartford's Hispanic communities have a history of struggling with Hartford Hospital and city government, calling for greater services for neighboring residents and more representation on key decision-making bodies. Hartford Hospital's efforts to engage in public outreach often seem to go unrecognized, while the origins of the hospital do not. For example, a local public health professional and community organizer told us Hartford Hospital was not the result of any public health initiative, but rather was "started with old WASP [White Anglo-Saxon Protestant] money . . . from the industrial era."

Facing decline in the early 1970s, the city's corporate leaders and the Chamber of Commerce formed a group called "Greater Hartford Process." The group's report, colloquially known as the "Process Memo," chronicled a sweeping urban planning project that sought to restructure the greater Hartford region, but ultimately failed to secure funding. Rojas (the professor at Central Connecticut State University) explained that Frog Hollow "was very poor and heavily Puerto Rican" at the time, and when someone leaked the memo, the Puerto Rican community, quite understandably, felt it was under attack. Rojas said the community interpreted the redevelopment plan as "Let's 'clean it out,' take that neighborhood over, and make it expand downtown." The memo explained that the failure of the Hartford Process to realize its initial goals required the group to take a second approach, rooted in a "triaging" strategy that called for the "containment of poor areas and their isolation from the downtown area."[30] The community staged protests to correspond with the opening of the city's new civic center in 1975[31] (see fig. 2.2).

The threat of major changes to community assets has been a central part of the history of the communities proximate to Hartford Hospital. Two years before the leak of the Process Memo, an eight-month-old baby named Rosa Maria Rivera was in distress, and her mother and family took her to both Mount Sinai and Hartford Hospital, but she eventually died in the back seat of a police car. The news made the front page of the *Hartford Courant*[32] (see fig. 2.3). The Hartford County Coroner determined the baby's death was due to acute gastroenteritis and dehydration, concluding that both hospitals demonstrated "some bad judgment" in not admitting the child. The subsequent malpractice lawsuit flagged the "substantial" language barrier as a partial cause, and the subsequent series of front-page news stories signaled the hospitals' failure to provide adequate services to the city's Spanish-speaking population.[33]

The stories of the Process Memo and Rosa Maria's death intersected in 1978, with the founding of the Hispanic Health Council (HHC), a community-based organization that describes its mission as "improv[ing] the health and social well-being of Hispanics and other diverse communities."[34] One of the group's early activities was fielding a survey, which revealed that a very high percentage of Puerto Rican women had been sterilized at Hartford Hospital. As the survey revealed, many of these women reported that their physicians had not clarified that the procedure, known in the Puerto Rican community simply as "la operación," was irreversible.[35] These revelations intersected with deep memories of other traumatic events—the U.S. government's reprehensible mass sterilization of Puerto Ricans both on the island and in cities such

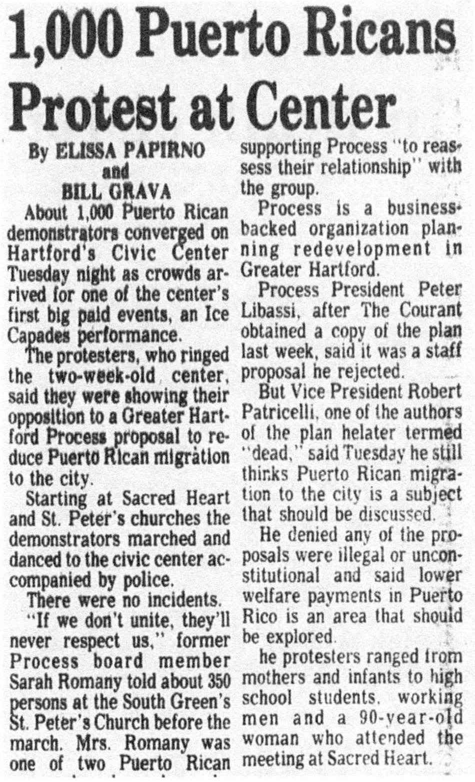

1,000 Puerto Ricans Protest at Center

By ELISSA PAPIRNO
and
BILL GRAVA

About 1,000 Puerto Rican demonstrators converged on Hartford's Civic Center Tuesday night as crowds arrived for one of the center's first big paid events, an Ice Capades performance.

The protesters, who ringed the two-week-old center, said they were showing their opposition to a Greater Hartford Process proposal to reduce Puerto Rican migration to the city.

Starting at Sacred Heart and St. Peter's churches the demonstrators marched and danced to the civic center accompanied by police.

There were no incidents.

"If we don't unite, they'll never respect us," former Process board member Sarah Romany told about 350 persons at the South Green's St. Peter's Church before the march. Mrs. Romany was one of two Puerto Rican

supporting Process "to reassess their relationship" with the group.

Process is a business-backed organization planning redevelopment in Greater Hartford.

Process President Peter Libassi, after The Courant obtained a copy of the plan last week, said it was a staff proposal he rejected.

But Vice President Robert Patricelli, one of the authors of the plan he later termed "dead," said Tuesday he still thinks Puerto Rican migration to the city is a subject that should be discussed.

He denied any of the proposals were illegal or unconstitutional and said lower welfare payments in Puerto Rico is an area that should be explored.

he protesters ranged from mothers and infants to high school students, working men and a 90-year-old woman who attended the meeting at Sacred Heart.

FIGURE 2.2. Newspaper articles of Hartford Hospital's relationship with the Hispanic community
Source: Hartford Courant, permissions granted.

as New York throughout the 1900s—reinforcing the lingering distrust of the U.S. medical establishment among Puerto Ricans, just as has been the case among African Americans.[36]

The HHC's mobilization against the hospital recalled and reaffirmed the successful mobilization of Puerto Rican political power against the city's Process Memo and redevelopment plan only a few years prior. Further, because of this history, many neighborhood residents continue to harbor suspicion about a range of Hartford institutions, with the hospital right at the center.

AURORA: A FRESH START WITH COMMUNITY ENGAGEMENT

The case of the recent opening of the Anschutz campus and the relocation of the University of Colorado Hospital differs from the histories in Cleveland

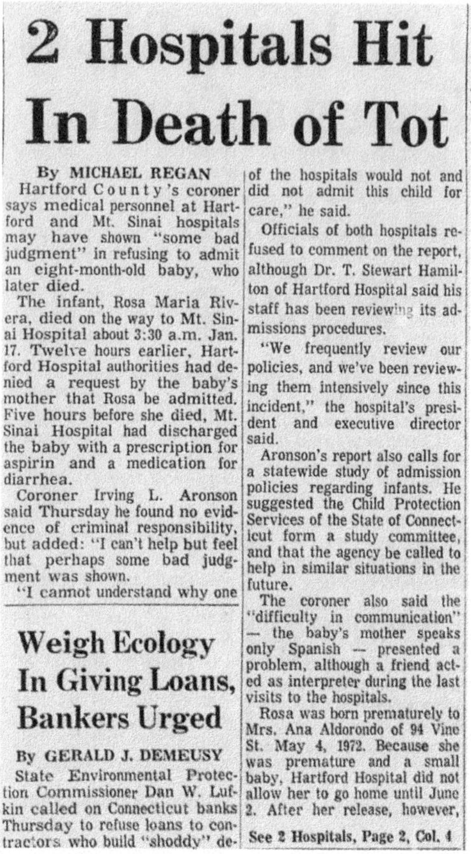

2 Hospitals Hit In Death of Tot

By MICHAEL REGAN

Hartford C o u n t y 's coroner says medical personnel at Hartford and Mt. Sinai hospitals may have shown "some bad judgment" in refusing to admit an eight-month-old baby, who later died.

The infant, Rosa Maria Rivera, died on the way to Mt. Sinai Hospital about 3:30 a.m. Jan. 17. Twelve hours earlier, Hartford Hospital authorities had denied a request by the baby's mother that Rosa be admitted. Five hours before she died, Mt. Sinai Hospital had discharged the baby with a prescription for aspirin and a medication for diarrhea.

Coroner Irving L. Aronson said Thursday he found no evidence of criminal responsibility, but added: "I can't help but feel that perhaps some bad judgment was shown.

"I cannot understand why one of the hospitals would not and did not admit this child for care," he said.

Officials of both hospitals refused to comment on the report, although Dr. T. Stewart Hamilton of Hartford Hospital said his staff has been reviewing its admissions procedures.

"We frequently review our policies, and we've been reviewing them intensively since this incident," the hospital's president and executive director said.

Aronson's report also calls for a statewide study of admission policies regarding infants. He suggested the Child Protection Services of the State of Connecticut form a study committee, and that the agency be called to help in similar situations in the future.

The coroner also said the "difficulty in communication" — the baby's mother speaks only Spanish — presented a problem, although a friend acted as interpreter during the last visits to the hospitals.

Rosa was born prematurely to Mrs. Ana Aldorondo of 94 Vine St. May 4, 1972. Because she was premature and a small baby, Hartford Hospital did not allow her to go home until June 2. After her release, however,

See 2 Hospitals, Page 2, Col. 4

Weigh Ecology In Giving Loans, Bankers Urged

By GERALD J. DEMEUSY

State Environmental Protection Commissioner Dan W. Lufkin called on Connecticut banks Thursday to refuse loans to contractors who build "shoddy" de-

FIGURE 2.3. Newspaper articles of Hartford Hospital's relationship with the Hispanic community
Source: *Hartford Courant*, permissions granted.

and Hartford, where deep memories are hard to reconcile or dislodge. A new beginning, however, can entail either a fresh start or a bungled first impression.

Tragic events can trigger community sentiments and action. The event most Americans associate with Aurora is one that residents would rather not be known for: a 2012 mass shooting at a local movie theater. One news outlet noted that media headlines tended to "name-check Aurora as the site of the massacre, rather than tying it to a Denver suburb."[37] Although the event horrified residents, it also fostered solidarity among Auroran communities and its institutions, and placed the city's new medical facility at the center of these bonds and emerging identity.

Several hospital administrators said they expected the hospital would be welcomed with a fair amount of goodwill when it moved to Aurora. These medical professionals see themselves as "out there saving lives and doing leading-edge clinical care." A high-level administrator at UCHealth explained that the initial assumption was that the diverse community "would automatically just love having us around," but in actuality it required continuous work to create a positive perception of the hospital among Aurorans.

For some residents, the new hospital complex brought hope of expanded healthcare access—a sentiment we rarely encountered in Cleveland and Hartford, where there was little optimism that the seemingly intractable barriers to healthcare access would change. However, not all Aurora residents felt as confident about the potential for the new campus and its various facilities to "do good." Discussing the area's immigrant and undocumented population, Carol said new Americans encounter too many roadblocks when they attempt to receive care. Institutions still operate within the same flawed, inequitable system. She remarked, "They help us the first time but when we try to continue, they ask us: 'What is your social security number?' or 'Where are your papers?' And we don't have them, so we cannot continue with the care." As a community that has been called Colorado's "top destination for immigrants,"[38] this is a major concern for local advocates.

Interviewees' fears intersected with the well-known local story about Eduardo Franco Ramirez that opened this chapter. The administrators we interviewed recognized that these well-known stories hampered their ability to foster working relationships with their neighbors. Many of these negative experiences were related to individuals not being able to access care because of their legal residency status or use of public insurance, or because of language incongruence. Some healthcare executives in Aurora lamented the fact that current state law creates a barrier to healthcare access for undocumented residents.

Stories like Ramirez's can be contextualized within the broader landscape of hospitals' responsibilities to communities, the histories of those specific communities, broader narratives about U.S. healthcare wherein hospitals do the bare minimum, and a wider national conversation about the treatment of undocumented community members. Once created, these deep memories shape local expectations, potentially for decades—sometimes despite some mixed attempts by hospitals to address past mistakes. For Aurora, a relatively short history could become a source of deep memory in a matter of years.

How Ideas of Place, Community, and Access Differ

The opening of the new Anschutz campus was an opportunity for hospital administrators to learn from their new community. The community hoped the hospital would listen. As Ellis, a local leader, said, hospitals need to "stop, and go on a real strong listening tour to understand that when you enter a community, fear and suspicion and all of these things naturally creep into residents' minds." Understanding and acknowledging the persistence of community memory is an urgent task for any anchor institution. But how, when, and to whom should hospital workers and administrators listen? The histories illustrated above offer keys for understanding the deeper memories that inhibit, impede, or enable productive and collaborative relationships, and healthcare access broadly.

The hospitals' treatment of immigration status offers an informative example. In both Aurora and Hartford, which have high concentrations of new immigrants, immigrant status is a major barrier to receiving healthcare. Residents reported forgoing healthcare, especially while the stridently anti-immigration policies of the Trump administration were in effect, because they feared exposing their status. One Hartford organizer said that when she visited a local family to help them troubleshoot their unsafe living conditions, their prior experiences with a landlord who threatened to report them to Homeland Security for deportation made them unwilling to approach the hospital for help. "It was a lesson for all of us," she concluded, "about people that have undocumented status, about why they don't go to the hospital until it's a real emergency. They feel they can't trust anybody." In Aurora, a Hispanic resident shared a story of her brother receiving treatment at University of Colorado Hospital—when he became agitated, a nurse responded by threatening, "If you don't calm down, I'll call immigration." Even though the hospital responded to the family's complaint by removing the nurse from the conflict, the resident believed that situations like these are the reason community members eschew healthcare initiatives.

These are merely two stories among many. Much of what residents expressed in our interviews reveals that a set of core ideas are contested when hospitals and communities meet. We found that stories around three core ideas—*place*, *community*, and *access*—form the foundation of community memory and shape how residents see hospitals in the present.[39]

PLACE

Despite significant contextual variation, our three hospitals share the impetus to expand their campuses into densely populated urban neighborhoods. While some development initiatives in Hartford, Cleveland, and Aurora sparked enthusiasm, others were met with indifference or even resistance among residents.

A 2015 survey indicated that 80 percent of U.S. hospitals were in an acquisition mode, seeking space for medical offices, outpatient surgery clinics, and health and wellness facilities.[40] Rather than seeing these developments as serving the needs of the community, residents often view them as working at cross-purposes. Hospital expansion, for example, is often interpreted as an unnecessary investment that overshadows the need to engage in community-level work.

Even worse, community members can perceive expansion as a threat. Residents, especially immigrant communities and communities of color, work to create a sense of place in their neighborhoods—building a durable place identity and fostering social networks that allow for inclusion and social mobility. Researchers of ethnicity and migration refer to these spaces as "ethnic enclaves."[41] Such placemaking might include the establishment and support of small, locally owned businesses (e.g., small grocers specializing in international goods, ethnic restaurants); increasing representation in local schools and government; and curating symbolic markers such as murals, flags, and signs espousing shared identities. From the community's perspective, this is a process of nurturing meaningful community assets.

Hospitals generally have a different approach to communities, focusing on physical rather than social geography.[42] In their own way, each of these institutions is involved in territorial positioning for greater market share. The Cleveland Clinic has grown from a clinic to a system, opening new outpatient and inpatient facilities throughout northeast Ohio, Florida, and more recently distant countries; Hartford HealthCare continues to grow throughout Connecticut; and University of Colorado Hospital's system, UCHealth, hopes to utilize the medical center as the foundation of its regional footprint. These different strategies make sense when considered from a population density perspective. Anschutz sits in a dense metro area that quickly becomes mountainous to the west and is sparsely populated to the north, south, and east. UCHealth appears to regard Anschutz as a destination—a vision complemented by the proliferation of hotels near the campus.[43] Hartford HealthCare continues to expand outward in concentric circles as it seeks to establish footholds within urban and suburban communities in the region. The Cleveland Clinic is also advancing outward, reaching farther and farther east and south into Ohio, for example, but is also rapidly developing outposts across the country and, indeed, the globe.

The placemaking of hospitals and the placemaking of communities often clash—one is based on the geography of regions and one is based on more of a cultural geography. Further, the asymmetry in power is not lost on locals.

Anita, a Cleveland city planner, reported that there is "some kind of agree-ment" between the city and the Clinic about the boundaries of what she re-ferred to as "Cleveland Clinic Land." Specifically, she said that the Clinic would not move south of Cedar Avenue or north of Chester Avenue, although she was unsure whether these boundaries were part of a formal arrangement with the city government. She insisted, "There's a master plan and the city's ad-opted it, so we're all going along [with it]." Thus, the "place" of the Clinic within and around its neighborhoods has been negotiated, formally and in-formally. Aspects of the informal negotiations are the subject of local mythology and speculation. Similar stories emerged in Aurora and Hartford. As shown in chapter 4, all three hospitals obtain, hold, and develop properties around their peripheries, prompting negotiations over what is, in Anita's terms, "Hart-ford Hospital Land" or "Anschutz Land."

In Hartford, a local realtor illustrated how hospitals can compromise or erase locations that serve as important parts of the community's place-based character. He described how the neighborhood received the news of Hartford Hospital's purchase and subsequent closing of a neighborhood funeral home, noting that it was a community "asset" and an "anchor" because it provided affordable funeral services to the neighborhood. "Now," he lamented, "they use it as a parking lot." As a long-standing institution, a hospital's business-driven decisions that appear to discount the value of established assets—whether those are individual homes or well-loved institutions—come at the risk of straining relationships.

The University of Colorado Hospital benefited, in some ways, from hav-ing a fresh start in Aurora's neighborhoods, even though the land itself had a long and consequential history in the community as a military installation. As a new institution, the hospital brought change both inside and outside its borders, altering the existing landscape in a way that jarred some neighbors. The hospital transformed the campus from a decaying military relic into an embodiment of the big business of American medicine.

The experience of being "on campus" differs markedly from that of being "in Aurora." The medical campus is largely secluded from the surrounding areas, and yet residents noted that the new campus changed the character of the nearby neighborhoods without improving the economic outlook of many of the residents. The residents we interviewed found this juxtaposition quite demoralizing.

Led by the Fitzsimons Redevelopment Authority, areas to the north of the campus, including the former Fitzsimons golf course, are now the site of rapid development that includes hotels and housing. To the south, a 10-block stretch of Colfax Avenue has morphed into an area that many Aurorans now view as "downtown" Aurora, though the medical center's direct role in this process is difficult to discern. Respondents reported sharp increases in rents, the construction of hotels and other accommodations for visitors, and improvements in the city's appearance resulting from updates to Aurora's once-decaying infrastructure.

Aurora highlights how hospitals and residents often see places differently. Hospitals are tied to place through history and explicit branding. Most envision themselves as essential parts of the city and local communities, and claim to celebrate their urban contexts as part of their ongoing efforts to celebrate themselves and their achievements in healthcare. Residents might see the value in the presence of these institutions within their communities, but also perceive expansion as a disruptive threat to local institutions and shared lives. Because hospitals fail to consult and genuinely collaborate with historically marginalized communities, these residents are often skeptical of their intentions and fear that their sense of place is under attack. There is, in other words, conflict over how hospitals and communities negotiate and respect place.

COMMUNITY

When asking hospital administrators and residents what community meant to them, we received very different answers. These answers were revealing, given that many hospital neighbors might not realize just how significant the term "community" has become in contemporary healthcare. As noted in chapter 1, for decades the Internal Revenue Service code has included language around hospitals' obligations to the "community," but this idea of "community benefit" has left many hospital neighbors wondering, "Whose definition of community?" For nonprofit institutions such as the three hospitals we are looking at here, the IRS code supports a more fluid approach to defining the physical boundaries of what constitutes a community, allowing institutions to serve "community" defined as either the patients they serve, a broader geographic region, or specific populations in need.[44]

Hospitals are currently looking to broaden their client-patient base by attracting medical tourists with state-of-the-art facilities, such as Hartford Hospital's new Bone and Joint Institute. Hospitals are reaching far beyond their immediate surroundings, across cities, states, regions, and even the world. To address the needs of this regional and global clientele, hotel capacity has become an important part of twenty-first-century hospital planning. The *New York Times* noted that "developers are seizing on the benefits of situating hotels near major medical centers, many of which are in hotel-starved outskirts."[45]

In Aurora, new hotels line the south side of Colfax Avenue, across from Anschutz Medical Campus, with plans for more on the north side. The Cleveland Clinic entered directly into the hotel business, opening two upscale hotels with almost 450 rooms (including a "Presidential Suite" we were told was
designed in consultation with the U.S. Secret Service to cater to world leaders
and VIPs), a move that turned heads and targeted a new revenue stream.[46]
The Clinic's hotels aim to host family members and recently discharged patients, if they can afford it.[47]

For residents, hospitals' competing visions and investments can be hard to
reconcile. Hospitals entering the hotel industry or focusing on increasing hotel room capacity on their perimeter, at the possible expense of amenities that
would serve the current residents of these neighborhoods, creates a sense that
these institutions provide excellent medical care to some while other populations do not receive the same benefits or level of attention. In all three case
studies, residents and local professionals echoed these concerns, namely that
their local medical center provided exceptional care, but only for others.

As stated in the introduction, these neighborhoods are hardly monoliths.
They are patchworks of groups from a variety of backgrounds, all of which
have their own histories and healthcare landscapes. It is also not lost on some
locals that certain neighborhoods received more attention than others. Georgia, who worked in community development at the Clinic, remarked, "Fairfax is where [the Cleveland Clinic] sits," and then said that she believed in
"taking care of home first and putting our best effort [in], but Hough would
be a very, very close second—that's the neighbor, the front door."

At the same time, hospitals do not merely define community along geographic or racial lines. In his study of the medical profession, Daniel Menchik
highlights how one hospital developed a new "bed management program"
that limited the number of beds to patients with private insurance by "essentially redefining its use of the 'community' to describe not neighborhood patients but those who would help the organization attain its goals for prestige."[48]
Their internal definitions of "community" may also be altered and redefined
in ways that are largely hidden from neighboring residents, even though, in
this particular case, the hospital used a public campaign to build local buy-in
while also limiting care to patients with illnesses that were prevalent in their
neighborhood, and discontinuing advertising campaigns in the local area.

While these definitional questions are potentially important in formal ways
(e.g., IRS code, bed management), it is still inevitable that hospitals will inter-
face with locals from many neighborhoods, not just the ones they've focused
their attention on. How these institutions engage with communities differently
can be quite telling.

ACCESS

Access to medical care, as well as other services that address social determinants of health, is closely tied to the contested ideas of place and community. Hospitals and their surrounding communities do not always share a definition of what constitutes access to healthcare.

A small business owner working near the Cleveland Clinic observed, "The first thing they ask you is 'Do you have insurance?'" A local politician recalled a constituent saying, "You could get shot outside in front of Cleveland Clinic's emergency room, but if you don't have a healthcare card, they're going to take you across town to the county hospital. They're not going to serve you." The politician acknowledged, "There's some truth to that." Mirroring the discussions of place and community above, a nuanced consideration of access reveals that physical proximity does not ensure access. Many interviewees in Cleveland perceived MetroHealth, with its emergency room just south of downtown Cleveland and other locations on the city's east side, as the place where elite institutions such as University Hospitals or the Cleveland Clinic funneled poor and uninsured Clevelanders in need of care.

Joe, who held a leadership role at Anschutz, said access in Aurora was the result of both the hospital's historical involvement with charity care, and the new expectations associated with being a new entity in a community. He acknowledged there is still a great deal of work to do to engage with local populations in an appropriate and effective manner. He noted, for example, that "one thing we brought to the table by moving to Aurora was access for the neighbors to that level of care that frankly they hadn't had before. There were obviously lots of challenges." For Joe, the depth of the disparities and other health challenges make it hard to assess expectations. He added, "In the eyes of some, it was never enough. I think the expectation is always higher in some eyes, and then what the availability can portend, and what the facility can provide." While Joe expressed pride in the charity care the University of Colorado Hospital accomplished in Denver, he added that they wanted "to meet the need, and the demand," after their move to Aurora.

In all three cities, health disparities concerned residents. Aurora's locals reported facing challenges in accessing specialty care despite the arrival of a major medical care center and hundreds of specialty providers in the last decade. The new campus brought hope of expanded healthcare access to some residents. One explained that, because it is "such a big university it makes people feel like they have a good place to go to. It seems like it has a lot to offer." While not all residents felt confident that they could use the services, some did. Jillian, for example, who directed a nonprofit, shared that "in general, having a local hospital is a good thing for neighborhoods," and then added, "certainly makes it easier, if nothing else, to get to an emergency room." Similarly, an Aurora resident stated that having a hospital nearby was helpful for providing healthcare access to a broad spectrum of residents. She commented, "There's a lot of low-income clinics; I know the hospital here provides services for uninsured people, and so do other hospitals in the area. I think that there's plenty of healthcare opportunities available."

A third group saw the medical center as offering different levels of access for different types of care. Anschutz may provide emergency care, residents explained, but few services were available for patients with specialty care needs. Bebe Kleinman, the director of an Aurora nonprofit, explained that despite living a "stone's throw" from the campus, residents and the grassroots workers helping them were saying, "We look up and we see these huge institutions, and I've made 42 calls and I can't get a dermatologist to deal with this issue." Anna, another Auroran, said healthcare was available, but not necessarily affordable. Referencing the growing number of costly urgent care clinics, she stated that service comes "at a high price," and added that many residents "wait until they are on their deathbed to go because they don't have insurance; they go to the emergency room." She continued, "In that respect they have the access, but it is costly access because of the bad healthcare," and concluded, "that doesn't make it a healthy city."

Perhaps most striking is that Anna's perspective doesn't seem entirely different from the perspective of someone who lives far from a large medical center. The considerations of residents living in the shadow of a world-class hospital are often no different from those of residents who struggle to access healthcare because of geographical distance from medical resources, such as rural Americans.

Contention and Trust

The contestation surrounding the terms *place*, *community*, and *access* undercuts efforts to improve health outcomes and, more broadly, hampers relationships between communities and their hospitals. Considering the importance of the concepts, and the significant differences of opinion and perspective on their meaning, the negotiation of these ideas should inform any future community work.

As scholars and activists pursue new ways of building relationships between institutions and communities, it is important to acknowledge that contention holds certain benefits for communities: it prompts communities to define place on their own terms, argue for seats at the table for residents, position themselves for access, and question the motivations of large urban institutions.

Interviewees repeatedly broached the issue of trust. Some residents raised concerns about what they believed were the long-term but private visions hospitals concealed from communities.[49] Others spoke of not trusting the U.S. healthcare system more broadly, which is a pervasive and historical phenomenon, especially along racial boundaries, as the chapter's epigraph from W. E. B. Du Bois shows. Healthcare workers, on the other hand, generally believed that they did good work, imbued with a Hippocratic moral foundation, and therefore the hospital was inherently worthy of trust.

Trust, as sociologist Teresa Gonzales rightly noted, is "rooted within systems of power and inequality," and it should not be surprising when mistrust emerges as communities—especially communities of color—interact with urban institutions that have development-oriented agendas.[50] Communities, she explained, hold and wield mistrust rationally as a tool for survival, dampening what they often see as unfounded hope to lessen the disappointment when promises go unfulfilled. Similarly, communities' "collective skepticism" of hospitals and other medical institutions can serve as an impediment to hospital-driven programming. Too often, mistrust is cast as a problem to be solved by the communities themselves, instead of a window into entrenched systems of power and long-standing histories of insult and disappointment.

Latino and Hispanic community members in Hartford portrayed their mistrust as just such a reaction to the history described above. While many administrators in Hartford had come to this reaction from residents, in Aurora, the community's stance of mistrust surprised administrators, who expected that being relatively new to the area and offering proximate high-quality and advanced care would automatically translate into a positive reception.

For Cleveland residents, mistrust in medical institutions had deep roots. As one Clevelander explained: "A fear of hospitals was instilled in me when I was young. Until recently, I hadn't been going to hospitals, and I was just like I'm gonna do what I gotta do. You'd say, 'Drink some orange juice; go to sleep.' That was the remedy for everything. Get you some vitamins, and rest. That's what you need. Because of the history of hospitals and the Black culture, you know." In this context, hospitals would need to address the larger historical context before residents would feel comfortable accessing an elite medical institution.

Others, like Mario, held a more nuanced perspective, noting that the persistence of health inequalities existed alongside better overall health outcomes. He recognized the outreach from the hospitals, believed that people were "being a whole lot more health conscious," and thought the medical campuses were "making a bigger impact." While Mario saw a causal mechanism by which the presence of a world-class medical center could improve local health out-comes, most of the residents we talked with merely hoped for this connec-tion, even if they couldn't quite identify specific improvements.

Communities are often unsure of what they can reasonably hope hospi-tals will offer to neighborhood residents. Despite the cynicism built over years of neglect, many communities of color seem to default to hope because there appear to be fewer available resources and institutions. Residents and those involved with organizations doing community development work often ex-pressed hope in similar ways. An administrator at the Cleveland Orchestra, which is part of the Greater University Circle (described in the previous chap-ter), for example, concluded, "We're going to have some quieter but more long lasting, and we hope, a transformational change in some of those neighbor-hoods." The reference to "quiet" reflected the sentiment among many organi-zations, including hospitals, that they are engaged in programming and plan-ning the residents may not always notice.

Importantly, as Gonzales explained, the expectation of trust by urban elites marginalizes dissent, invalidates local sentiments and histories, and devalues reasonable concerns. Indeed, the residents we interviewed in Aurora, Hart-ford, and Cleveland showed that mistrust serves as an important resource in keeping communities of color vigilant. This instrumentalism explains a Hough resident's assessment that newer residents will have more trust in the Cleve-land Clinic while "a lot of the older residents will not." In many ways, the Clinic needs to create a fresh start by attending to long-standing open wounds while also managing new opportunities to engage with a new generation of residents. Starting over, however, does not mean forgetting.

Conclusion: History in the Present

Understanding barriers to healthcare utilization and population health im-provement in a community requires an awareness of the local stories sur-rounding hospitals' presence in and expansion into neighborhoods, their pol-icies determining who can receive care, and their mission and reputation. For many reasons, recent activities aimed at improving public health outcomes do not seem poised to ameliorate long-standing pervasive mistrust, which can stunt access to healthcare and harm health outcomes.

There is considerable evidence that trust in healthcare systems drives health-care utilization.[51] Medical institutions can shape trust in a variety of ways, from influencing local norms and the sociodemographic composition of commu-nities to improving access.[52] Hospitals, however, must do this work through the lens of the specific histories of institutions and communities. We argue that these community histories are critical to understanding local culture, which is a strong "neighborhood effect," alongside other social determinants of health. As this chapter shows, however, an adequate appreciation of the role memory plays within communities highlights key concepts that clarify the complicated interplay of institutions and communities.

The current findings show that mitigating the present barriers related to limitations in the formal structures of healthcare delivery is necessary but ultimately insufficient for addressing historical problems. Locals' comments illustrate that working with surrounding communities requires hospitals to take a longer view. The harm institutions have caused to local communities is well documented. Merely recognizing the impact of past practices, even if they differ greatly from current approaches, is a great step, but is also insufficient.[53] The data suggest the need to push this project further. In particular, there is good reason for residents to fear that hospitals will fail to acknowledge their complicity in systemic racism, with locals dismissing hospitals' seemingly antiseptic urban development initiatives as little more than public relations efforts. Indeed, these development initiatives may even intensify the very policies they purport to correct.

It is important to recognize the powerful role local histories play in shaping health beliefs and perceptions of care. Chapter 3 does this by considering different institutional approaches to contested definitions of place, community, and access. The major actors who work in health-oriented community development programs—advisory board meetings, public health department initiatives, nonprofit collaborations, medical institution programs—often seem to assume that initiatives that improve conditions in the present also heal historical wounds. However, as both the current data and prior research have shown, this type of oblique engagement undercuts programming in the present. Likewise, hospitals have not actively cultivated a greater understanding of local perspectives in their efforts to promote access to care. Considering this oversight, we suggest that storytelling and explicitly historical work might be keys to promoting access to care and fostering collaborative interventions between hospitals and communities.

Direct historical reckoning is a heavier and more costly lift. Without it, however, medical institutions are unlikely to remedy race- and class-based disparities in either their clinical spaces or their surrounding neighborhoods. Such failures will only further compound mistrust.[54] The assessments of residents of Aurora, Cleveland, and Hartford presaged the observations of commentators during the COVID-19 pandemic, where entrenched histories of discrimination and distrust intersected with issues of access and prevention, especially with regard to vaccine hesitancy.[55]

3

"What's Your Total Commitment
to the Community?":
Explicit and Implicit Hospital
Development Strategies

The vibrancy of the surrounding area is certainly important to us as we recruit staff,
faculty, and students, and for the patients and families who come to our hospital. There
is no denying we have an important institutional interest in this area . . . But having a
more livable, vibrant community is good for the residents of this area. We are eager to
demonstrate to young and old alike our commitment to this project.
RONALD R. PETERSON, former president of Johns Hopkins University[1]

As keystone urban institutions, hospitals can support the vibrant mix of their
neighboring communities or disrupt existing dynamics. Many hospitals explicitly evoke community engagement in their mission statements. For example, David Portillo (manager of the Strengthening Neighborhoods Program
for Denver's Funder's Committee for Civic Participation) explained that the
Anschutz Medical Center follows other medical facilities, such as the Mayo
Clinic, in presenting engagement as something they "owe the community."
Portillo said these institutions need to communicate their "total commitment
to the community." A professor familiar with the dynamics of Cleveland's institutions and communities explained that there are consequences for hospitals if they do not make strides in community development beyond caring
for emergency medical needs. "If you don't understand that," he commented,
"you're gonna be besieged." Statements like these were fairly common. Given
the growing expectation for hospitals to undertake this work, it is understandable that administrators would acknowledge the importance of community
engagement.

Whereas chapter 2 illustrated the distinct histories of these three sites, we
can now look to some of the common strategies through which hospitals engage in community development. Across this chapter, and continuing on into
the following two, we take note of similarities while also flagging important
differences. This chapter takes a wide view of hospitals' engagement in community development, moving beyond the public relations work, sponsorships, and
free health screenings provided by hospitals. While the formal tax requirements

for community benefit are discussed in chapter 1, community development is a broader term that includes multi-sector collaborative enterprises focused on changing a neighborhood's symbolic, cultural, and/or economic landscape.

Save for occasional economic impact statements and highly structured community benefit reports, few reliable frameworks exist to shed light on the impact of hospitals' community development.[2] The following sections examine both the implicit and explicit strategies of development projects, as well as their potential effects on communities, including gentrification and displacement.

Anchor Institutions and Community Development

In the broadest sense, community development is an undertaking in which public, private, and nonprofit organizations work to "strengthen the economic, physical, and social environments of low-income neighborhoods."[3] The primary focus of community development is to improve the quality of life for residents within a given geographic region, often loosely defined. Development initiatives can achieve this goal by growing local capacity for leadership development and resident empowerment,[4] and connecting neighborhood institutions with organizations outside the area.

Community development can target education improvements, affordable housing programs, and home-buyer incentives; foster small business development; improve access to fresh food and groceries; bolster health clinics; increase property values; nurture social capital; create amenities; or attract additional investment. Such work varies depending on the local context, as communities differ significantly in their social and organizational ecologies.[5] Various actors—elites, residents, and local activists—and institutions compete, collaborate, and realign to engage in official and unofficial strategies to change their communities.

As shown in chapter 2, hospitals and communities often perceive their relations quite differently. While communities increasingly pressure anchors to invest in their neighborhoods,[6] residents have mixed feelings about the resulting changes. Community members in all three of our cities saw hospital development work as engineering the physical, social, and economic landscape in both welcome and unwelcome ways. Hospital administrators, on the other hand, knew their institutions used their extensive power largely for the public good. Georgia, a Cleveland Clinic employee with a role in community development, remarked that the Clinic can serve as an "anchor for the whole state," but they also want to work with neighborhoods like any other anchoring institution. In the same breath, she said she knew that a multibillion-dollar organization is different from a church, school, or library. She continued, noting that she "comes to the table" with neighborhood stakeholders with an important caveat: "We're the biggest and we try not to be the biggest, if you know what I mean, and let everyone have a voice."

Richard, who works with health nonprofits nationally, including organizations near the hospitals we studied, reported that communities "have never gotten their fair share of dollars or resources" from anchor institutions. A better understanding of development sheds light on just what does, or does not, constitute a "fair share." This chapter analyzes community development in terms of explicit and implicit development strategies. This approach clarifies initiatives and illuminates why they deserve both criticism and praise.

The Explicit Community Development Agenda: Hire, Live, and Buy Local Programs

Hospitals are fond of promoting community development programs that cohere around a catchy promise of being "local" in hiring, staff living arrangements, purchasing supplies, and more. Neighbors' assessments of such programs are mixed. Communities sometimes see these strategies as tangible improvements and other times see them as extremely superficial.

"HIRE LOCAL": OPPORTUNITIES AND UNCLEAR PIPELINES

The President and CEO of the Connecticut Health Foundation, Patricia Baker, explained that because U.S. health coverage is largely tied to employment, "health and well-being are directly related to jobs." Kenneth, a Cleveland nonprofit worker, also focused on the importance of jobs, summarizing the

TABLE 3.1. Examples of "Go Local" programs

Hire Local	Anschutz Campus institutions adopted a "Hire Local" program developed by the Greater University Circle Initiative in Cleveland to a) coordinate hiring across institutions, b) develop entry-level jobs for locals, c) reevaluate hiring policies that serve as barriers to entry for residents, and d) establish a job hub to assist in navigating application processes.
Live Local	The City of Hartford, Southside Institutions Neighborhood Alliance (SINA), the Chamber of Commerce, and area employers launched the Hartford Home Ownership Incentive Program, which offers up to $10,000 per applicant to incentivize employees of the community's anchors to purchase homes in downtown Hartford.
Buy Local	The Cleveland Clinic's "Supplier Diversity Advisory Council" identifies local suppliers as part of an effort to meet institutional diversity goals (e.g., incentivizing larger majority-owned companies to identify parts of their supply chain where they can hire smaller, minority-owned businesses).

community's perspective succinctly: with the hospitals, "many people just want jobs."

Hospitals often carry urban employment sectors on their backs, and some can tout their status as a significant economic engine of the city. The Initiative for a Competitive Inner City reported that hospitals create more inner-city jobs than any other economic sector, and healthcare is the largest employment sector in 77 of the largest 100 urban areas in the U.S.[7] Indeed, the three research sites are the largest employers in their respective cities, according to the U.S. Department of Labor. As of 2022, the Clinic employed 32,000 people, the entire Anschutz campus employed 25,000, and Hartford Hospital employed 6,000.[8]

Further, hospital positions are often excellent jobs. Lilly Marks, Vice President of Health Affairs for the Anschutz Medical Campus, told us their jobs often pay more than the median household income in the surrounding neighborhoods, and include health insurance and retirement benefits.[9] Urban public hospital jobs are also accessible for neighborhood working-class populations; about two-thirds of hospital jobs require less than a bachelor's degree.[10] And while many jobs are entry-level positions, they can provide a foothold, create "job chains" for other residents, and help new hires "climb the ladder" through skills training and credentialing.[11] According to Heidi Gartland, Vice President of Government Relations and Child Advocacy for Cleveland's University Hospitals, such programs nurture "pride" among the staff and "increase employee engagement" in communities.[12]

Administrators at all three hospitals expressed some level of commitment to local hiring. Hartford has historically taken a passive approach. Emeritus Chief of Surgery at Hartford Hospital, David Crombie, noted that staffing changed in tandem with demographic changes in the neighborhood in the late 1960s and early 1970s. As the ED began admitting more Hispanic and Latino patients, the hospital's hiring reflected those changes, primarily in "nursing services, clerical services, [and] record keeping."[13]

Our other two cities, however, adopted more intentional "hire local" programs. The program in Cleveland began when the Cleveland Foundation wanted to "shift the economic paradigm" (in the words of a local nonprofit CEO) by developing local worker-owned cooperatives and, in 2008, sponsored a research trip to Mondragon, Spain, with representatives of University Hospitals and the Cleveland Clinic.[14] Based on what they learned, the University Circle institutions launched the worker-owned, nonprofit Evergreen Cooperatives, which provides stable jobs for locals and goods for the hospitals. The Evergreen Cooperatives launched Evergreen Energy Solutions and Green City Growers—making 100 employees across all cooperatives (almost half of whom were members/owners), who earn an average annual income of $23,450

($5,000 more than the area's average annual income).[15] In 2018, the Evergreen Cooperatives assumed the management and operations of the Clinic's laundry, doubling their employees.[16]

Cleveland's programs gained enough recognition that planners in Aurora took notice. Lilly Marks at Anschutz recalled that the idea of being an anchor institution was "new" to leaders on the medical campus. Fred, a physician and administrator, said a delegation of university, hospital, and city officials headed to Cleveland to learn more. According to a former Aurora city councilor, a jobs program was one of the first points of agreement; she explained that "the one thing that the campus could do [was] to create income" that would stimulate homeownership and improve health outcomes.[17] Anschutz quickly adopted the program. Laughing, Fred remarked, "We even stole the name 'Hire Local.'"

Establishing cooperatives, however, is a relatively rare practice in the U.S. We identified five additional strategies hospitals used to increase hiring rates in communities: coordinating campus hiring efforts,[18] targeting specific jobs for local hiring, changing hiring policies, launching job search and application assistance programs, and developing K–12 health education programs.

First, like the Clinic, the Anschutz campus institutions coordinated their hiring efforts. Justin, who worked in family medicine at Anschutz, said the different campus entities created an "employers working group" to be "intentional about local hiring." The group focused on diversity needs, including the growing local refugee population.

Second, the working group focused on positions that Justin described as "practical ways to get people in the door": housekeeping, janitorial, food and nutritional services, patient services, and front desk and lower-level administration. Marks said they targeted "800–900 jobs across Anschutz that only require a high school diploma."

Third, hospitals evaluated their hiring policies, especially those likely to block many neighbors from applying. For example, a Clinic administrator explained that while they maintain a policy to not hire smokers, they now hire people with criminal records to address the vicious cycle of criminalization and unemployment. In Aurora, hospitals adopted new protocols so human resources departments would give nearby residents strong consideration, including adding a "hire local checkbox" to capture local zip codes on applications.

Fourth, hospitals addressed access. Former Aurora mayor Ed Tauer and Melvyn Colón, Director of the Southside Institutions Neighborhood Alliance (SINA), both conveyed residents' frustration that their hospitals' job applications were posted and submitted online. Residents in all three cities reported limited internet access and online competency, and hospital job ads made the process even more challenging: despite efforts to streamline, each Anschutz facility had separate processes, titles, and positions. Jimena, an Anschutz neighbor, said community pressure led to the 2018 establishment of a physical off-site job hub one block from the Anschutz campus in a space donated by the Aurora Strong Resilience Center.[19] Similarly, University Hospitals, the Cleveland Clinic, United Way, and other entities took part in a program called "Welcome to Fairfax" that was administered by the Fairfax Renaissance Development Corporation. Expanded considerably in 2015 and 2016 with support from the Clinic, the program facilitates "soft skill development including building technology skills and access, financial literacy, referral to supportive services and training and internship opportunities."[20] A member of Fairfax Renaissance said the group's goal is to "recruit, screen, and train residents for employment with many employers, Cleveland Clinic being one of them."[21]

Finally, programs in Cleveland and Aurora sought to improve the jobs pipeline through formal relationships with local schools. In Cleveland, Courtney noted that attempts to "get more underrepresented students into the health field" are asking a lot of a "struggling" school district. The University of Colorado Hospital developed a "learn local" program, focusing on creating pipelines for K–12 Aurora students who express an interest in the health sciences. Collaborative initiatives include programs that bring "targeted groups" of high school students to the Anschutz campus as well as "Lunch and Learn" meetings where medical and other health professions students can talk with high school students about careers in healthcare and "how to get there."[22] Two administrators at Anschutz said they worked to create a pipeline from the schools to the Community College of Aurora to help local students obtain jobs in five identified areas: patient services, food and nutrition services, environmental services, certified nursing assistant, and medical assistant. They explained that this meant "starting with GEDs and going all the way through," including getting certifications for new immigrants who "might be medical professionals in another country but they can't get a job here."

"LIVE LOCAL": HIRING LOCALLY
AND ENCOURAGING HOMEOWNERSHIP

Matthew Desmond's Pulitzer Prize–winning book *Evicted: Poverty and Profit in the American City* is a stunning portrayal of what happens when people don't have a home.[23] Because of the negative effects of housing insecurity, housing has become one of the most widely and well-researched social determinants of health, credited with shaping the disparities in health outcomes seen across U.S. cities.[24] Poor housing is associated with many risks (e.g., financial stress, delays in seeking healthcare, exposure to toxic materials, and proximity to

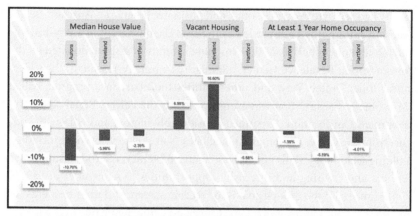

FIGURE 3.1. Housing characteristics in hospital neighborhoods relative to city averages
Source: American Community Study 2018 (5-year estimates).

social stressors such as food insecurity and violent crime), and thus housing is both a critical dimension of neighborhood stabilization and a cornerstone of community health. Many interviewees, both inside and outside hospitals, flagged lagging homeownership rates and housing insecurity generally as a concern in their respective cities, while also acknowledging that most hospital employees lived far outside these neighborhoods. "Live Local" programs that increase household incomes and neighborhood stability are the flip side of the "Hire Local" coin.

Unlike Cleveland and Aurora, Hartford has a fair amount of vacant housing stock in the downtown area, including neighborhoods surrounding Hartford Hospital (see fig. 3.1).[25] We were lucky to spend some time with Cary Wheaton, who was the Executive Director of Hartford's Billings Forge Community Works before her passing in 2021. Wheaton estimated that Frog Hollow had at least 400 abandoned buildings. To illustrate, she paused the interview, directed us to a window, and pointed to a building next to her office and three others across the street. The hospital, she believed, should be compelled to "address that most of their professional workers don't live in the community, or even in Hartford."

Kerri Provost, a local archivist and writer we spoke with over coffee at a Frog Hollow café, concurred. She expressed disappointment over Hartford's wealthiest employees disproportionately living in the suburbs—particularly the hospital's employees, who she believed had markedly different responsibilities than those who worked in other industries. She concluded, "I want the people who can do the lifesaving to live closer to where they work—that's a little more important than the person running the insurance company." Both

Wheaton and Provost tied residence to the missions of anchor institutions, especially the hospital.

Ivan Backer, SINA's first director, noted that the amount of cheap housing stock around the hospital made a good early programmatic target for their organization because many of those working in the lower-level workforce could reduce transportation time and costs while also tightening the connection between the hospital and the community. SINA's current director, Melvyn Colón, still characterized Frog Hollow as a "neighborhood of tenants," and Hartford's Director of City Planning and Economic Development concurred, saying the area's less-than-10-percent owner-occupancy rate is a significant concern and "an area to focus on [for] opportunities for owner occupancy."

David Crombie recalled that when SINA reached out to support Hartford Hospital's housing program, the hospital lent their design and engineering staff to help renovate neighborhood houses; the team developed 83 units across 13 Frog Hollow buildings. In 2012, the City of Hartford, SINA, the Chamber of Commerce, and area employers launched the Home Ownership Incentive Program to incentivize employees of the local anchors to purchase homes downtown. Through the program, if an employee purchased or rented a home nearby, they received a $10,000 grant for housing assistance.

Cleveland and Aurora had similar programs. Funded by several anchors and administered by the Fairfax Renaissance Development Corporation, Greater Circle Living offers employees from one of three dozen area organizations a forgivable loan for down payments on houses, one month of rent, or (if they already have a home) exterior renovations on homes within the University Circle area.[26] In Aurora, a 501(c)(3) called Live Where You Work offers employees financial incentives of up to $17,000 as long as they remain in a full-time position and stay in residence for at least five years. Co-founder Sally Mounier, who was also a former member of the Aurora City Council, said the costs of these programs are "chump change" for the nine partner institutions.

"BUY LOCAL": ATTRACTING AND LEVERAGING SUPPLIER BUSINESSES, NURTURING DIVERSITY

In 2016, the Democracy Collaborative, a national nonprofit focused on local economic development strategies, released a toolkit for hospital/community development.[27] The organization noted that while health systems spend over $340 billion annually on goods and services, "many of those dollars do not reach populations facing the greatest health disparities."[28] Distressingly, the group also found that less than 2 percent of health system purchasing comes from businesses owned by minorities or women.

Given local histories and the social and economic patterns characterizing U.S. cities generally, it is unsurprising that decades of disinvestment and deindustrialization have made it difficult for anchors to source needed products locally.[29] COVID-19 highlighted this dilemma: hospitals commonly rely on goods from not just other cities and states, but international companies; however, the pandemic slowed and even shut down supply lines for personal protective equipment, ventilators, and other equipment.[30]

"Buy local" programs required creative thinking about how to reward existing businesses and support new ones. As a hospital administrator remarked, these programs seek to "improve the economic viability of the community," keeping suppliers close while simultaneously infusing capital directly into nearby neighborhoods to stabilize local employment, create closer relationships between hospitals and communities, and promote supplier diversity.

Differences in scale between hospitals and local businesses often led to power imbalances and other incongruities. Melvyn Colón described Hartford's decades-long economic decline as hampering "buy local" efforts. He showed us a large red binder kept in the SINA offices. "We used this," he explained, "to record all the businesses in the area, what they produced, and what their capacity could be." Colón said he brought the binder to meetings with the anchors, but noted, "The scale of their need, however, is more than what most of our local businesses can really manage." Marcus McKinney, Vice President and Chief Health Equity Officer at Trinity Health of New England, had worked with SINA in the past and confirmed this assessment. He estimated that Connecticut Children's and Hartford Hospital spent one-quarter to one-half billion dollars on goods, and added that few local businesses could meaningfully service these institutions.

In an attempt to traverse these roadblocks, Cleveland got creative. An economic developer who worked for the city explained that their office incentivized hospitals to attract or keep suppliers local. The city recognized that hospitals needed to "keep their source of bandages and sterile instrument kits" local, so they asked hospitals, "Why don't you use the power of your contracting ability to bring this company in with these jobs so that we could help people get them?" These companies then signed long-term contracts to move to the city, and City Hall worked to find locations and economic incentives.

ASSESSING "GOING LOCAL" INITIATIVES

Have these programs worked? The results are mixed. Hire/Live/Buy Local programs sometimes appear to be more important to hospitals for what they signal than for what they deliver.[31] "Going local" is intuitively attractive as a mode of improving community relations, but the underlying economics are

TABLE 3.2. Change in healthcare employment from 2009 to 2018, comparing hospital neighborhoods with areas immediately surrounding them

		2009	2018	% Change
Aurora	City average	16.1%	18.8%	+12%
	Contiguous	14.4%	18.5%	+28%
	1st Ring	11.6%	15.6%	+34%
Cleveland	City average	24.2%	25.6%	+6%
	Contiguous	45.8%	40.1%	−12%
	1st Ring	32.1%	43.4%	+35%
Hartford	City average	26.4%	29.5%	+12%
	Contiguous	27.1%	24.3%	−10%
	1st Ring	25%	35.3%	+42%

Source: Based on ACS 2018 (5-year estimates).

unclear. After all, in a rapidly growing-yet-consolidating healthcare landscape, the effects of community investment might not go beyond counterbalancing historical policies and current trends.

We asked for employment data on hiring locals to gauge the success of "hire local" efforts, but received limited information. About 2.8 percent of the Clinic's employees hailed from the surrounding neighborhoods.[32] Hartford's SINA program, which facilitates employment in neighborhood institutions, placed 56 residents at Hartford Hospital, and 15 at Connecticut Children's so far. Lilly Marks said the programs at Anschutz hired 670 employees from targeted zip codes to date (140 of those were in 2017).[33] Isaac, a physician and professor at the University of Colorado, looked at local employment, as well as health indicators and outcomes from community health survey data, and found little change in the years after the campus opening. "Unfortunately," he concluded, "we haven't seen [improvements] as robustly as one might like. There are jobs out there, but they're not going to the community."

We gleaned some evidence on employment from survey data. The areas around the hospitals have changed. In the census tracts immediately surrounding the Clinic, there was a 12 percent drop in employment in healthcare between 2009 and 2018, and a 35 percent increase in the next series of census tracts. In Aurora, the change in healthcare employment near the hospital significantly outpaced the change in the city (see table 3.2).

Meanwhile, vacancy rates around the Clinic increased 14 percent over this period, while the vacancy rates in the city also increased, but only by 5.5 percent. Vacancy rates in the areas around Hartford Hospital improved significantly and to a greater degree than in the city overall, while the vacancy rates in the areas around Anschutz kept pace with the city overall (see table 3.3).

TABLE 3.3. Change in vacancy rates from 2009 to 2018, comparing hospital neighborhoods with areas immediately surrounding them

		2009	2018	% Change
Aurora	City average	9.1%	4.3%	−53%
	Contiguous	13.6%	6.5%	−52%
	1st Ring	8.5%	4.3%	−49%
Cleveland	City average	19.1%	20.2%	+5.5%
	Contiguous	24.6%	28.1%	+14%
	1st Ring	23.7%	24.2%	+2%
Hartford	City average	15.6%	14.8%	−5%
	Contiguous	21%	14.3%	−31%
	1st Ring	23%	11.8%	−48%

Source: Based on ACS 2018 (5-year estimates).

Interviewees generally agreed that hospitals must focus their commitments on applicants. Deborah, formerly of the Cleveland Foundation, said she received feedback from residents that they still didn't "feel welcome" enough to apply. As Marks explained, jobs programs are "very labor intensive, expensive, and the actual return isn't great yet." Emerging initiatives and partnerships might do well to address building trust, because inconsistent and ineffective hiring and education programs can frustrate and further alienate locals.

The general neighborhood consensus about "live local" programs is that anchor institutions must invest more to meet demand. Interest in each of these programs exceeded capacity. Since its launch in 2008 (and relaunch in 2012), Greater Circle Living has served 459 Clinic employees. Among the program's participants, 35 percent used funds to purchase a home.[34] In Hartford, Colón described the housing program as a success. Each year, contributing organizations had exhausted available subsidies for participants. So far, 29 employees from Hartford Hospital, 12 from Connecticut Children's, and 7 from Trinity College have taken advantage of the program.[35]

Connecticut Children's Community Relations Manager Stephen Balcanoff said their live local program "raises the value of the properties over time, and it's there where we [as institutions] can help." Indeed, Colón reported that these new tenants represented "somewhere in the neighborhood of $250,000 a year added to the tax rolls." Characterizing one aspect of the neighborhood perspective, longtime resident and community organizer Hyacinth Yennie commented that the benefits of these programs are more than financial: "If you own a home and can walk to work, you're going to pick up trash when you see it and, you know, call the cops if you see a problem . . . You have a stake in the neighborhood." To varying degrees, these "live local" programs are innovative and promise to contribute to the successful stabilization of housing in these cities.[36]

Among these local programs, the "buy local" program in Cleveland has had the greatest success. Of the Clinic's $2.2 billion of procurements in 2017, $227 million—10 percent of the total—went to vendors in the City of Cleveland.[37] Further, Cleveland isn't just using hospitals to attract businesses; they are addressing diversity and problems by scaling their programs to ensure that they have an impact. The Clinic established a Supplier Diversity Advisory Council, which convenes quarterly and comprises both institutional personnel and community members. Alex, a Clinic employee, described the project's aim as assessing the institution's needs and then working with local businesses to determine whether they have the capacity in production to "bridge that gap." He offered several examples—construction, HVAC, street signage, printing— of places where the suppliers with whom the Clinic contracts can also be part of a broader diversity effort. When the Council cannot find local vendors who can handle the Clinic's needs, they turn to a mentor/protégé program. The supplier diversity program incentivizes larger majority-owned companies to "carve out" or "de-bundle" a part of their supply chain for smaller minority-owned businesses, and then "take those vendors under their wings to show them the ropes." Careful facilitation of these relationships is crucial for Alex because he knows that "people have a tendency to do business with people whom they know and who they feel comfortable with." Notably, the Clinic's "diverse spending" declined in recent years, from $158 million in 2018 to $130 million in 2019 and $73 million in 2020.[38] Programs like this one provide pathways for minority-owned businesses through mentorship, logistic connections, social networks, and entry into these institutions' massive procurement chains.[39] They require, however, a great deal of effort and commitment to implement and maintain.

Overall, these programs lay the groundwork for bolstering communities where socioeconomic deprivation drives poor health; in addition, such programs may foster relationships that were damaged in previous eras when hospitals hoarded resources. An examination of the dynamics of these efforts reveals that while clear roadblocks impede their progress, there are also signs of promise.

The Implicit Urban Development Agenda:
Perimeters and Corridors

"Hire/Live/Buy Local" initiatives get a good deal of attention, but they are only a part of what hospitals do in their communities. Hospitals are also important cogs in what urbanists call growth machines. Growth machines are linked urban organizations that shape land value through capital and symbolic investment but are rarely investigated as key factors in this perspective.[40] We identified two interlinked strategies wherein hospitals serve in this capacity: *securing the perimeter* and *corridor vision*. While they receive less attention than the programs described above, taken together these strategies have profound ramifications for neighborhoods.

The use of more tactical language to describe this second type of activity is deliberate, as many in the surrounding neighborhoods see hospitals and anchors as invasive forces. For example, one healthcare nonprofit executive observed there is a "horrible" and "long history" of urban institutions treating neighborhoods as "spaces to create parking lots or new towers." Further, as shown in chapter 2, neighborhood residents track developments, though their knowledge ranges from a loose understanding of broad moves to specific details of acquisitions and expansions and, less so, at the level of strategy. While administrators were eager to promote the programs discussed in the first half of this chapter, they were reluctant to talk about this second type of initiative. Despite, or perhaps because of this hesitancy, a discussion of these underreported activities is crucial.

SECURING THE PERIMETER:
LAND GRABS, FLASHPOINTS, AND EYESORES

Continuing the Hartford walking tour we described at the start of chapter 1, a visitor could head north up Washington Street, keeping Hartford Hospital to their right. They would soon arrive at the eight-story Connecticut Children's Medical Center, built in 1996. SINA's founding director Ivan Backer reported that some of the campus's growth has been on properties they "already owned." Specifically, he mentioned a nursing home owned by the hospital, which the hospital demolished to build a children's hospital—technically a separate entity but very much a part of the medical campus in the eyes of the community.

When the visitor reaches "Presidents Corner"—the intersection of Washington and Jefferson Streets—their view is of parking lots and boarded-up buildings. Kerri Provost divulged that, as a "nerd" and a member of a Neighborhood Revitalization Zone (what Connecticut designated as partnerships between residents and their municipal government for neighborhood development), she would research who owned abandoned properties at the city assessor's office and then report the owners. She paid attention to hospital-owned lots, which included a boarded-up building that once housed 40 low-income residents. Nearby, the visitor will spot the former location of a beloved funeral home that a local real estate agent, Luis, who worked extensively in the area, called "a great community asset"—it is now a parking lot owned by the hospital.

Walking through the hospital campus, down Seymour Street and among patients and medical staff, the visitor passes through the Bone and Joint Institute. The Institute's Director and Chief of Orthopedics, Courtland Lewis, described it to us as "a learning laboratory," and asserted that orthopedics is "probably the number one moneymaker for hospitals everywhere right now." When we toured the facility, we learned the physicians there do dozens of elective surgeries a week, as well as "a whole bunch" of trauma surgeries. Tucked behind the new institute is a brick building that used to house Peter's Retreat, a supportive housing facility for people living with complex medical issues including HIV/AIDS, which was operated by Hands On Hartford, a nonprofit human services agency. Kate Shafer, who worked at Hands On Hartford, said the organization sold the building to Hartford Hospital, enabling both entities to expand their services to the community: Hartford Hospital was able to realize its goal of establishing the Bone and Joint Institute, and Hands On Hartford was able to establish the Center for Community, where it continues to provide food, housing, and health support to Hartford residents.

These expansions and acquisitions create flashpoints in these relationships, and stoke concern and folk-hypothesizing about what land the hospital will acquire next. A few blocks to the north, Billings Forge's Cary Wheaton indicated that this was a reasonable fear, given what she saw as the hospital's history of "property grabs." She even had a list of places she expected hospital administrators had on their radar. Provost also sensed there was a broader plan at work; her comments echoed Wheaton's view: "They'll buy a property," she said, "sit on it for a long time, and then strip it down to build some other facility we don't want." This assessment draws on the community's opinion that primary care services do not meet needs and specialty care isn't for them. Ron Pepin, a planner for the City of Hartford, said the hospital has "50-year plans" for development they keep private, and historically has been "very reluctant" to engage with the surrounding neighborhoods.[41] When we asked Courtland Lewis about this appraisal in a top-floor conference room of the Bone and Joint Institute, he confirmed the plan, explaining that funding was being secured for the next capital investment. He declared, "I'm telling you straight out. They absolutely have plans to create a . . . flagship for the health system [and] it's evolving."

For Aurora, the history of the University of Colorado medical campus being blocked from expansion by their downtown Denver communities shows

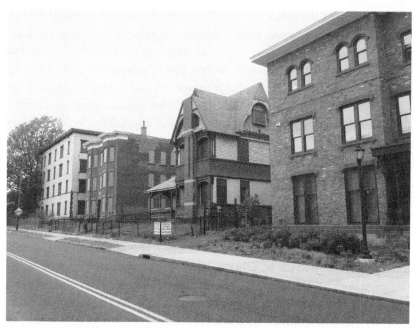

FIGURE 3.2. Three vacant buildings owned by Hartford Hospital on Jefferson Avenue across from the hospital, next to the new Hartford Hospital Community Health clinic (Photo by Wynn)

there are limits to a hospital's acquisitive aspirations. The neighborhoods surrounding the Anschutz campus presented a major opportunity. Most respondents, both inside and outside the hospital, described the surrounding area as
the site of run-down hotels, pawnshops, and what a former politician called
"home-based pharmaceutical distribution and sales," all of which contrasted
starkly with the desired image of the new medical facility.

Former mayor Ed Tauer (who served from 2003 to 2011, after his father,
who served as Aurora's mayor from 1987 to 2003, retired) believed that, from
the city's perspective, the area's redevelopment was warranted: property values needed to rise to counter the medical facility's property-tax-free nonprofit
status. He maintained that it's the government's job to "generate taxes when
you can," and one of the best ways to do so is to provide services for out-of-
towners: patients, families, and conference attendees. Tauer explained, "You
have to develop hotels for conference centers." Judith, who worked at the Children's Hospital, characterized new hotels as partners who make it possible to
house the families of children receiving care on the medical campus.[42]

Isaac said the new campus had already "come close to running out of room,"
and Councilwoman Mounier said future expansion and development plans
will be directed north, to the Montview neighborhood. Three government of-

ficials involved in city planning—Joy, Kelsey, and Carl—reported that the Fitz-simons Redevelopment Authority's strategies had raised concerns among their constituents. Joy observed that the Authority "slowly just started buying houses and houses and houses and then eventually they bought [the entire neighbor-hood] because they were outgrowing their space." These officials noted that their office is "trying to control how much of [development north of Mont-view] can be housing." The essence of the debate was clear from these inter-views: Should the need for growth eclipse community needs?

The Cleveland Clinic's local reputation echoes the perceptions of hospitals we witnessed in Hartford and Aurora; however, we also recognized signs of collaboration, seemingly in response to decades of high-profile tensions and negotiations.

In the 1970s, when the Cleveland Clinic considered moving to the suburbs, the institution decided, instead, to double down, "launching the expansion of the 1970s and persuading the governors and trustees that all available real es-tate adjacent to the Clinic should be acquired."[43] An urban planner in Cleve-land said that more recently, the Clinic "bought up a ton of property and it's driven up prices like you wouldn't believe." Courtney, an employee at Metro Health, added that the Clinic's history of purchasing and demolishing build-ings in the area fueled distrust among residents. In addition to discussing these more aggressive moves, however, some interviewees mentioned that the Clinic has at times collaborated with local residents.

Like Hartford's Neighborhood Revitalization Zones, Cleveland has Com-munity Development Corporations, or CDCs, which are nonprofit entities es-tablished under 501(c)(3) of the federal tax code and exist to improve conditions in specific neighborhoods, focusing on housing and economic revitalization. Shelly, who worked for a nearby CDC, said she noticed a change in tone, ob-serving that while the Clinic was reticent to share long-term expansion plans in earlier years, the development department now works with her CDC and they "talk constantly" about properties, eventually finding answers that work for both parties. She concluded, "That's huge."

Shelly pointed to the Clinic's revival of an old building in the neighbor-hood. The Clinic wanted a space to offer off-campus services, while the Fairfax Renaissance Development Corporation wanted to save the historic Langston Hughes Library (see fig. 1.5 in chapter 1), which was meaningful to the local Black community. The $5 million project restored the building, which now houses Senior Outreach Services, an agency that serves the health needs of older Black neighbors, from nutrition classes to yoga, as well as an office where the Clinic provides free physicals, immunizations, screenings, and healthcare navigation.

COMMUNITY DEVELOPMENT VIA HEALTH TECH,
ARTS, AND LEARNING CORRIDORS

Across all three sites, neighbors, stakeholders, developers, and residents talked
about corridors: Frog Hollow has the Learning Corridor, Hough has the Knowledge Corridor, and Aurora was planning an arts and culture corridor. These developments constitute the second way hospitals operate as growth machines—
by shaping and creating physical and symbolic bubbles around their campuses and expanding their borders.

Corridors are planning initiatives that center on land use, co-locating similar services proximate to urban institutions and resources such as transportation, infrastructure, and even culture along narrow geographic areas—like tun-
nel vision for development. Businesses are, in fact, wary of relocating to areas
that do not offer sufficient amenities and restaurants.[44] A Cleveland city planner
commented that corridors are an attractive strategy because people increasingly prefer to work in less-institutionalized spaces—areas without parking garages or security checkpoints—rather than in the more traditional office spaces
in the city's downtown. A representative for the Cleveland Clinic reinforced
the community's perception of how hospitals approach their neighborhood
when he said, "The current road to campus goes through neighborhoods that
people don't want to go through," and then added that corridor work would
"help staff and patients get to the hospital faster."[45]

Cleveland's Health-Tech Corridor stretches along Euclid Avenue, with a
transit line running alongside it (a bus route christened the "HealthLine," established through a deal with University Hospitals and Cleveland Clinic in
2008), connecting the city's "two downtowns": downtown and University Circle.[46] Kurt, a Cleveland nonprofit leader, said both major infrastructure and
investment projects in-fill the area with businesses and industries wanting to
be close to both urban hubs.

Jeff Epstein, Director of the Health-Tech Corridor, reported that once the
Cleveland Foundation was involved, it convened the University Circle leadership and city hall. In Epstein's words, the organizations said: "Look, this is
the condition of the surrounding neighborhoods. What are you doing about
it?" Epstein said he was inspired when the initiative was launched in 2010 and
described his goals for the corridor as threefold: to create a "destination" for
technology and health technology businesses, to stimulate real estate development, and to nurture the cluster of companies. This required, he explained,
"a bit of evangelizing" and "a bit of marketing." Epstein said the corridor coordinates some activities around jobs, housing, and procurement. In addition,

the Clinic has a tech and innovation incubator facility near the eastern end of the strip, generating businesses in hopes they will establish themselves nearby. He envisions both "high-end" and affordable housing coming soon but for now is focusing on attracting and maintaining middle-income housing, hoping to keep it "a pretty mixed-income community." Shelly, who works for a nearby community development and planning nonprofit, characterized the corridor as helping existing businesses improve and expand as well as attracting new talent.[47]

We observed a different nexus of development at the southwestern edge of Hartford Hospital's campus: the Learning Corridor, mentioned at the start of chapter 1 (see fig. 1.6). The 16-acre campus was launched due to a 1996 Connecticut Supreme Court ruling determining that state agencies needed to place desegregation of the city's schools "at the top of their respective agendas."[48] Stakeholders initiated educational reforms, including Open Choice school programs, part-time exchanges, and the development of the Learning Corridor. The Hartford Board of Education was in dire straits at the time—charter schools were at risk and the city's education governance was in crisis—making a partnership between schools and the SINA institutions one of very few options. A contaminated former bus depot site in need of remediation was selected for the corridor due to its proximity to Hartford Hospital and Trinity College, and the $220 million endeavor was funded through a combination of state and anchor institution investments.[49]

The corridor geographically and symbolically bridges Trinity College and Hartford Hospital and stitches together the neighborhoods around both institutions. Community leader Hyacinth Yennie described it as "SINA's biggest project." Yennie was the president of Hartford Areas Rally Together (HART), a nonprofit intermediary between the institutions and the surrounding neighborhoods. Nearby residents met regularly at a local church, and Yennie said that they felt the project attended to local needs, highlighting how certain aspects of the plan were changed due to residents' input—she explained that HART argued to keep a strip of houses on the south end, and "didn't want to even approach" the owner of the gas station at the site "about selling the property" because residents felt he was a good community member, hiring kids for summer jobs and teaching them business. Planners agreed with HART.

When the Learning Corridor opened in 2000, it gained national attention.[50] In addition to four magnet schools (a Montessori school, a middle school, an Academy of Math and Sciences, and the Greater Hartford Academy of the Arts), the corridor was to have a Boys and Girls Club, a job training facility, and a social service agency at the site. Kim Stroud, Director of the Arts at the Greater Hartford Academy of the Arts, noted there was also supposed to be a community health center, called The Commons, to attend to students' healthcare needs. According to respondents, the plan was for Hartford Hospital to staff the facility, which would serve as a connection point with the neighborhood, in the initial stages.[51] The Commons, however, never materialized, and Stroud described it as an example of the "magical thinking" of the overly optimistic early days of the project.

There was also talk of corridors in Aurora. To the north of campus is a public golf course that closed in 2017 and is currently in the process of development. The property is owned by the Fitzsimons Redevelopment Authority, an entity directing the commercial development of the former Army hospital; the development was originally called the Fitzsimons Life Science District but was later renamed the Fitzsimons Innovation Community. The Authority planned for the site to have several bioscience facilities, apartments, and hotels, as well as an elementary school, middle school, and high school. When talking about an area to the south of the medical campus, Ellis, who works with an Aurora-based nonprofit, said, "The bottom line is that basically there's a vision for that whole corridor to be turned into an arts district with condos and apartments all the way down."

Corridors are a logical strategy for urban development; however, they can create jarring economic, social, and cultural change, and introduce stark contrasts. For some community members, focused development looks like unequal development. The results might be visually dramatic, but they might also be traumatic for those displaced by the new additions. Aurora, in particular, has experienced very unequal development, an outcome that is not lost on the area's residents.

Institutional Growth, Gentrification, and Displacement

In the face of anchor-driven development, communities can feel squeezed between the left hand of feel-good "local" programs and the right hand of more implicit urban development programs.[52] Unsurprisingly, gentrification—the process of wealthy people moving into a poor or working-class neighborhood—and the resultant displacement of the area's original residents cast a shadow on conversations with interviewees inside and outside hospitals.[53]

Data from Matthew Desmond's Eviction Lab show that all three cities we studied were well above national averages regarding evictions (see fig. 3.3). Aurora's eviction rates were initially lower than the national average but then skyrocketed in the aftermath of the economic downturn, increasing from less than 1 percent in 2009 to 9.1 percent one year later (while the U.S. average rose

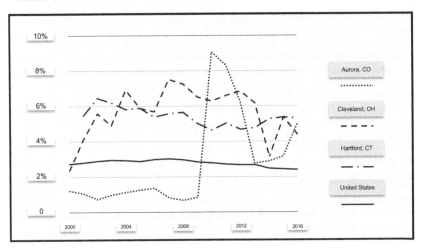

FIGURE 3.3. Evictions in Aurora, Cleveland, Hartford, and the U.S.
Source: Data from Eviction Lab, Princeton University.

slightly, from 2.91 to 2.95 percent).[54] In 2016, Hartford's eviction rates were 3.39 percent above the national average, Aurora was 3.18 percent above the national average, and Cleveland was 2.19 percent above.

Administrators expressed some awareness that homeownership programs and development projects along corridors could displace locals or lead to real estate speculation. For example, because potential Hartford homebuyers seeking "Live Local" grants had to work with SINA, we asked Luz Conde, a former SINA employee and longtime resident who had worked with the homebuying program for years, how the program worked. She explained that SINA carefully vetted applicants to ensure they were not exploiting the program for speculative purchasing:

> My process for that was "Do you want to live here?" If you don't want to live here, don't buy a house here. Because we don't want you. The reason SINA and the hospitals started the homeownership project was to stabilize the neighborhood. . . . Speculators try to buy quickly. But, in having to work with us, they understood from the beginning, this is about stabilizing the neighborhood. Live in this house for 15 years. You don't want to be here, you gots to go. And some people just left. They didn't want to be part of the program. Other people were committed. They were from the neighborhood. They wanted to buy in the neighborhood. They're staying here. I thought that was important. When I'm talking to people about housing, I say, "You don't want to meet your neighbors? No? Then this project is not for you. If you want to meet your neighbors, this project is for you." It was amazing. Most people stayed.[55]

While hospital administrators had some concerns about development leading to the dislocation of longtime community members, Colón remained "convinced that the only way [locals] can stay in a neighborhood is by buying a property" and believed that "buy local" programs would create a mixed-income community. "We don't want a community of all affluent folks," he noted.

Regarding the development of the corridor in Cleveland, Jeff Epstein said that "the goal" of business development was to "strengthen the communities around us and create mixed-income communities without leading to massive gentrification." Many residents regarded gentrification as a nearly inevitable byproduct of hospital growth. We heard this concern from Clevelanders such as Kenneth, who works with a nonprofit in Hough, and offered a stark view when he concluded that these developments were "changing neighborhoods" without any benefit to residents. In contrast, Cynthia, who works at an addiction services group, commented that while there is certainly a perception of the Clinic as a "monster that will eat our community," she felt city neighborhoods were "vibrant, strong," and had "enough land [to] welcome new people coming in, new ideas, new business, new homes." Development can't, she said, "do anything but make our community better."

Data from Cleveland's "live local" program offers insight into how these programs shape neighborhoods. Researchers who studied Greater Circle Living found that the demographic profile of program participants (38 percent white, 23 percent African American, 22 percent Asian, 16 percent other, and 1 percent Middle Eastern) diverged markedly from the residential makeup of University Circle neighborhoods, some of which were as high as 92 percent African American.[56] Further, the program attracted University Circle employees with a variety of salary ranges, although participation was higher among those with annual incomes of less than $50,000 or $50–75,000 than among those making more than $75,000.[57]

With a less robust "live local" program, we heard less anxiety about displacement and gentrification in Hartford. Residents, politicians, and activists alike pointed to a surplus of good but vacant housing and expressed hope for new residents and development. Billings Forge's Cary Wheaton, for example, was sanguine about a potential influx of new neighbors. Commenting on gentrification, she said there was "room to grow" without displacement, and that Hartford "would be lucky to have that problem on the horizon."[58]

The story in Aurora was quite different and is worth closer attention. Initially, Aurora's new facilities and employment opportunities sparked a great deal of enthusiasm. Lois, a Latina resident, had a positive response to the hospital's transformation of the area: she said that before the hospital relocated, the "run-down, high-crime" area was "riddled with motels, prostitution, and drug dealing," and she was grateful for new businesses. "From what I've heard," she remarked, "everyone was happy about it."

Some of our interviewees, however, were not happy with the changes in their communities. Mario, a longtime Auroran, said the once-affordable neighborhood held great social and economic value for those who lived there. Pointing to the cheap hotels, ethnic stores, and rental properties, he explained that those businesses were vital for low-income "families who have grouped themselves in that area."[59] Ellis recognized the "great" benefits of the campus while also complaining about the declines in low-income, affordable, and bridge housing. He noted that as developments reach into old neighborhoods where Hispanic families have owned their homes for generations, there will be a "tipping point" and an eventual "clash." City officials couldn't help but concur: a former Aurora council member said the city's housing market had "mushroomed" since the founding of the campus,[60] and former mayor Paul Tauer acknowledged that Aurora's immigrant and refugee communities had likely experienced displacement.

Allen, a lawyer, observed that medical students are flooding Aurora's affordable housing market. While recognizing that students may come from low-income backgrounds, he said families in the neighborhood "could use those spaces." Kevin, a community organizer for underrepresented groups, offered a series of rhetorical questions to illustrate how these changes were affecting these groups: "Who is then going to have inflated property tax values? Can they stay in their home? Or if they just get a fantastic offer, and figure this is their chance to make some money and move out? . . . It's displacing folks. We're seeing many people leaving the state because they can't afford a place to live." Neighborhood residents felt the pressure in a variety of ways: Allen said he'd seen landlords push out recent immigrants by remodeling and increasing rents for new tenants; a group of Aurora city planners noted that they had observed speculative buying around the hospital; and interviewees passed along secondhand accounts of residents receiving frequent phone calls with offers to sell their homes.

Development's influence on older Aurora added to the strain. Locals did not respond well when a trailer park across the street from the hospital campus was demolished to make room for new hotels and shops that would serve healthcare providers and patients. In another example, a 92-room hotel on Colfax Avenue, the King's Inn, was arguably an eyesore, but some city residents called it home for over 15 years. When it was sold in 2017, a transaction widely regarded as the result of pressure from Anschutz, the new owners doubled the rates, threatened tenants with eviction, and kept the building in "filthy" condition.[61] Many long-term residents were displaced almost overnight. In response to public outcry, the city ultimately earmarked $80,000 in tax revenue from legal marijuana sales, plus another $200,000, for a "flexible housing fund" to help residents relocate; the fund has served as the centerpiece of a broader commitment to addressing the city's persistent problem with homelessness and housing insecurity.[62] Former mayor Ed Tauer said it was "incumbent on the city" to find housing for these folks, and caseworkers approached "every single person," especially if they had school-aged children. He was "shocked" at how few of the hotel's residents took advantage of housing programs, and hypothesized that financial circumstances or prior convictions limited participation.

Aurorans mentioned other community amenities and cornerstones—a dress shop, a bakery, restaurants—that were closed or under strain. Tauer recognized that replacing a grocery store that catered to low-income, new immigrant, and refugee families with a new hotel "took a service out of the community," although he also commented that he wouldn't miss many of the buildings surrounding the medical campus.

Mario, a South Aurora resident, observed that these resources helped folks like him feel this was "where we belong." When he used to walk down the street, he told us he would see generations of families. "Then," he added, "suddenly, we saw micro-breweries pop up, new restaurants, bike shops, and the neighborhood changed completely." Mario said the hospital "went quickly from a symbol of hope to just another way that we are pushing the least fortunate in that part of Aurora out." To illustrate these changes, he pointed to a new Panera Bread chain restaurant on the former site of the grocery store.

Frank Anello, who is Co-Founder and Executive Director of Project Worthmore, a local nonprofit serving Denver-area refugees, and sits on the ward's zoning committee, argued that these activities are "100 percent gentrification." He remarked that the city "talks about diversity as an asset," but saw the medical center as "pushing on the community." Fred, who works in hospital/community relations, said the Aurora city government doesn't have the "will [to stop] the reality," adding that politicians are "in love right now with all the development going on."

At all three sites some residents ascribed ill intentions to hospital administrators and saw hospital-related developments as having unintended negative consequences (e.g., higher rental rates, speculative purchasing, and the dislocation of poorer, working-class, and non-white communities); Aurora, however, could have expected such outcomes. A North Aurora–based city councilmember who served during the planning and implementation of Anschutz identified what she considered a major stumble in the planning process: because student housing was not addressed until late in the game, a negative impact on the existing housing market was almost inevitable. Few developers would have begun such a large-scale construction project in parallel with a development project like the medical campus, preferring to wait until the completion or near-completion of the project. That timing, however, paired with the 2008 economic downturn, meant that the housing developments only took shape well after the medical campus opened.

Hospital administrators were aware of the potential for displacement. Sallie Hanfelder, former Director of the Eastern Colorado VA Health Care System, which included the Edward Hines Jr. VA Hospital, said the administration was aware their new facilities attracted new employee-residents who "buy houses and increase the cost of living." Hanfelder saw the potential for these developments to push out immigrant communities, noting, "sometimes you have to be careful what you ask for." When we raised these concerns with Lilly Marks at Anschutz, she noted that their next phase of development, to the north of campus (beside two new hotels and a few restaurants), included "fairly high-end apartments" for faculty and students (see fig. 1.3 in chapter 1). A group of Aurora city planners described the new housing as an attempt to provide more parking and retail space but also to "control growth before it gets out of hand" by having housing options for faculty and students as well as a range of housing for workers of "all types."

These efforts, however, arrived late. Some Aurorans believed gentrification and displacement had fatally eroded the area's new American community, and the eviction data for Aurora certainly suggest this is the case. Aurora lawyer Allen said the changes decimated the community's cohesiveness. Many residents moved away. Alexandria, a community health worker in Aurora, said that their programming has had to change to "meet the needs of displaced patients." Frank Anello of Project Worthmore confirmed that they had "lost a lot of our community, [who were] moving to other states, Indiana, Iowa, Kentucky, and moving in to areas where it is more affordable, [where there are job opportunities like] meat processing plants." For those who remain, the once active, lively, and diverse community is now, in the words of the former director of a downtown nonprofit, "invisible."

"We Don't See the World the Same Way": Different Voices on Development and Communication

At the beginning of this chapter, we introduced Georgia, who worked in community development at the Cleveland Clinic and described the Clinic as having the "biggest" voice in the area and the state of Ohio overall, even though it tried not to dominate conversations around development. Residents reported feeling that anchors weigh in heavily—and sometimes too much—when it comes to community decision-making. The point is a reminder that public relations personnel must often tread lightly, balancing their goal of promoting work taking place within the hospital—which is often touted in a celebratory way that is a familiar part of hospital advertising—with the more complicated and often sensitive work they do in communities. While public relations can be an effective tool for improving hospital/community relations, hospitals must take care to ensure that perceived space, or even contradictions between the implicit and explicit agendas, doesn't inflame anger among neighborhood residents.

In the three communities, development occurred at a pace and scale that seemed more reminiscent of a slow-moving natural disaster than a human-made one. We interviewed dozens of residents in a variety of positions in and around hospitals, and they overwhelmingly indicated that they felt powerless in the face of anchor- and hospital-fueled developments. As a result, communities were understandably skeptical of any hospital decisions. That hospitals are famously tight-lipped about their plans only exacerbated residents' apprehensiveness. SINA director Melvyn Colón's assessment of Hartford Hospital as "a little hard to read" echoed the thoughts of others in the communities surrounding the hospitals.[63]

City governments empathized with the community's perspective. A planner at the City of Hartford, Ron Pepin, said he tries to get the city's anchors to be "more open, more integrated, more connected to the community," but he has to balance those interests with being "more flexible in zoning controls [because] they're not gonna be able to continue to expand their campus internally." Ron explained that he wants communities to have greater access to the services hospitals provide, and sees "parts of the facility as an amenity" for their neighbors. He continued, noting the hospital's agenda "doesn't always jibe" with the community's, not just with respect to planning individual buildings, but development broadly considered. "We don't see the world the same way," he said, "and they keep their [plans] close to the vest."

Hospitals keeping their development plans secret made sense—for them. Releasing information might lead to land speculation or give property owners bargaining leverage that would cost the hospitals and might even spark a wave of evictions. The result, however, was that the communities were left to read tea leaves, only learning of plans and developments long past their necessary decision points. Anchors and their affiliated growth-oriented organizations facilitated a community-wide understanding among residents, hospital employees, and nonprofit leaders alike, all of whom reported that homeowners often "sit" on vacant buildings rather than investing in them, hoping land values will trend upward.

And yet these communities were vocal about wanting to play a greater role in what happens in their neighborhoods, and voiced pessimism about the hospitals' willingness to listen to community needs. For example, Laura Ann Frey, Program Manager at the Village Exchange Center in Aurora, described hospital-led community meetings held in or around the medical campus as follows: "They come in and want your opinion and they will give you a gift card for $5 or something. We gave you our opinions. Let's see you implement them." She characterized the hospital's response as, essentially, "No, we are just studying what is happening." The nature of hospital-led listening sessions can stoke an already-palpable belief among residents that hospitals are not interested in their input, and that such sessions are an end in themselves.

Other neighborhood voices centered on economic inclusion. For example, Luis, the Hartford real estate agent, said that hospital redevelopment efforts marginalize Hispanic and Latino community members, blocking them from participating in, and profiting from, the transformation of their own communities. He observed that smaller local developers who want to invest in the area "can't compete," concluding, "a local guy who wants to turn things around here can't afford it. They're priced out." Community leaders, he said, felt similarly: "They try to figure out how they can benefit and synergize their activities, in some type of economical insurance of this area." Unfortunately, Luis reported that these leaders hadn't had much success. As Chris Stocking, a Cleveland dietitian and community health advocate, asked, "How will we make these institutions more inclusive?"

For a possible answer, we turn to the case of Cleveland, which strongly and explicitly emphasizes anchor-driven community development, as well as wealth building and economic inclusion, as key goals. The Evergreen Foundation and the Clinic's supplier diversity initiatives remain models for hospitals seeking to increase economic investment in neighboring communities. With respect to housing and gentrification, an Auroran lawyer, Allen, said hospitals and city politicians have options they choose not to pursue. They should, in his estimation, advocate for affordable housing and support laws that curtail gentrification by creating land trusts and communal land-holding programs: community-owned properties held as collective assets. He complained that "it is just not happening. The city council and the mayor, I don't think they are open to the idea."[64]

Richard, the nonprofit worker we quoted above, had other ideas. He wanted "Hire," "Live," and "Buy Local" programs to address income insecurity and housing shortages. He also described "leverag[ing] the institution's assets to build meaningful community wealth in the low-income communities that they serve." Strategies could include not just supplier diversity but employee ownership programs, community land trusts rather than traditional home-ownership models, and "a place-based investment strategy that really identifies the gaps in the ecosystem around wealth building." And perhaps these efforts will catch on. In Aurora, Judith said the medical campus, including the children's hospital where she worked, was "starting down the path of potentially creating a significant fund that gets leveraged to flip some of those hotels [near Anschutz] into a different ownership structure and change their use and provide better housing options for low-income families."

For Jillian, who worked for an Aurora nonprofit after-school program for marginalized communities, the city was "like a giant ladder." But who gets to climb this ladder? Hospitals, or the surrounding neighborhoods? Our research clearly shows that if a hospital-driven development is to be perceived as successful, local residents need a greater share of the opportunity. An interviewee at the Billings Forge farmers market summarized this perspective when she concluded her comments on economic inclusion by evoking the old political slogan: "Nothing about us, without us."

Conclusion: What Is Meaningful Change?

On the ground, it is impossible to have a comprehensive view of development. David Stradling, a professor of history who coauthored an important book about Cleveland, described the challenges of development in the city, explaining that residents "wouldn't necessarily notice any positive change if they themselves didn't get a job." He added that while new institutions and businesses are being built, if they don't serve the community, "then the change is quite literally meaningless" to residents.

Our examination of these sites revealed how hospitals engage with communities in both obvious and subtle ways. Sometimes hospitals reported high levels of openness to collaboration in their communities. For example, the Clinic's relationship with Fairfax is more positive and cooperative. The relationship with Hough, in contrast, is marked by a tense past and its current dynamic is focused more on real estate and corridor development than community collaboration.

As Stradling emphasized, without an understanding of how anchors work in these communities, it's hard for locals to have enough information to distinguish between what is "about" them and what hospitals are doing "without" them. The dual approach taken in this chapter—reviewing the hire/live/buy local framework that hospitals and other anchors use to understand community development, and conducting an urban sociological analysis of this development—offers a more holistic understanding of the relationships between hospitals and their communities. This sheds light on the reach and limits of hospitals' aspirations and the effects these initiatives have on communities.

While a full accounting of these dynamics is beyond the scope of this book, this chapter's framework provides guidance for scholars, activists, locals, and administrators alike. Chapter 4 examines the effects of these development strategies with an eye toward the specific places in which new interactions occur, in other words, the social sites of exchange, or in the terminology of the academic literature, "contact zones."

4

Healthcare in the Contact Zone:
Unconventional Spaces, Institutional Changes,
and Communities of Color

> Care is an embodied experience for both the caregiver and receiver . . . Theories of
> habitus, perception, verbal and non-verbal communication, and performance are use-
> ful here to deepen our understanding of care as a form of "doing" or a mode of "acting"
> on different levels and in different registers: more verb than noun.
> ARTHUR KLEINMAN, *The Lancet*[1]

The 1990 documentary film *DiAna's Hair Ego* featured a South Carolina hair-
dresser partnering with a local physician to address the growing HIV epidemic.
Frustrated by the lack of outreach in African American communities, DiAna
built a grassroots movement to provide sex education, distribute condoms, and
destigmatize discussions about safe sex in her hair salon.[2] This initiative and
similar partnerships use trusted environments to improve health outside formal medical spaces. Research has shown that upstream prevention efforts that
include non-medically-trained community members can play a role in improving health outcomes for even the most difficult-to-treat illnesses.[3] This lesson
has spread beyond the medical field to political efforts—inspired by the success of grassroots efforts like DiAna's, the Biden administration fostered partnerships with local barbershops to help increase vaccine uptake during the
COVID-19 vaccine rollout.[4]

Hospitals and medical centers are expanding their focus beyond the clinic,
too. Partnerships with trusted neighborhood residents seek to identify local
health problems and devise new ways to address them. Indeed, in recent decades medicine has made strides in thinking creatively about the sites and
modes of engagement through which health promotion is staged. Recent efforts have led to a proliferation of new sites for prevention and clinical care,
from mobile mammography units to pop-up vaccine clinics at fairs to street
medicine, which seeks to meet unhoused individuals where they are to provide medical services.[5]

Hospitals also aim to offer more than clinical care, seeking new opportunities to address social and economic issues that hamper community health.
Accordingly, this chapter explores the spaces in which hospitals and commu-

nities meet—how these spaces are changing, what they mean for the medical field, and how neighbors relate to large anchor institutions and leverage needed community health improvements.

As the preceding chapters show, race plays a central role in this relationship. Zoe, a high-level program director involved in community health in Cleveland, described the overall perspective of the healthcare profession as trying to stay in a "relatively narrow lane." She asked us rhetorically, "Who are we to be thinking about racism? Who are we to be thinking about poverty? Who are we to be thinking about food security?"

Zoe said her colleagues are slowly realizing that addressing racism is "absolutely" their role. She characterized the American Academy of Pediatrics' stance in making policy statements on food security and poverty as a recent and "progressive" development, as was the Cleveland Clinic's position on addressing nonmedical needs in the surrounding communities. Race, she concluded, is an inescapable factor on the ground, calling local disparities in asthma and infant mortality "staggering" and "totally unacceptable."

Zoe explained that she believes solving healthcare problems requires a "new understanding" that bridges economic, racial, and spatial barriers. Her assertion animates this chapter's discussion. But where should this "new understanding" reside, strategically and programmatically? How can stakeholders arrive at a common understanding in the spaces where neighborhood communities and hospitals converge and sometimes even clash?

What's a Contact Zone? Beyond the Emergency Department

Anthropologist Mary Louise Pratt used the term "contact zone" to denote places where different cultures "meet, clash, and grapple with each other, often in highly asymmetrical relations of domination and subordination."[6] This term facilitates the analysis of how different communities interact in public transportation, cafés, museums, and other public sites, in both small towns and highly segregated and unequal urban environments.[7] The term is apt for our research sites because of the abiding demographic and economic gaps across the hospital/community divide.

Encounters in contact zones are meaningful, but contact is not always positive and can, in fact, exacerbate inequities.[8] An examination of contact zones can help identify the barriers to effective or ethical contact—including segregation, limited opportunities for interaction, language differences, and mistrust—that have historically undermined community/hospital relationships. Uneven awareness of these inequalities and histories has prompted health systems to invest in social work and healthcare navigation, in different ways and to varying degrees. At the same time, although social workers, navigators, and community health workers are becoming mainstays of healthcare workforces, it is not clear to what extent such services can address deeper structural inequities and overcome systemic barriers.[9]

Emergency departments (EDs, sometimes colloquially referred to as "emergency rooms") are often the primary point of contact between a hospital and the surrounding communities, particularly poor residents. EDs play an outsized role in both the imagined and actual versions of U.S. health policy, from providing uninsured Americans minimum emergency care (including the "surprise" bills patients receive) to providing care for undocumented and documented immigrants. Scholars have studied EDs extensively, noting their sociological significance for understanding community-level vulnerabilities and the complexities of community health generally, all of which lead to a perceived overuse of EDs. Over the past decade, scholars have criticized this concern with overuse, calling for a more humanistic understanding of why patients visit EDs and what they experience there. At the same time, urban hospitals continue to use EDs to serve the poor, actively as well as passively. Because of existing mistrust, undocumented people and those involved in the criminal justice system might avoid certain hospitals for fear of deportation and being reported to local authorities, respectively.[10]

Suffice it to say, EDs are suboptimal primary contact points between hospitals and their communities.[11] Therefore, with an eye to atypical and unconventional healthcare spaces, the rest of this chapter highlights the hospital/community contact zones outside EDs that emerged from the interview data, all of which were sites of both meaningful encounters and significant barriers for hospital staff and neighborhood residents alike. While the encounters we describe are certainly not the only ways communities and hospitals interact, focusing on the interactions, dynamics, and outcomes in these contact zones offers important insights into the city/hospital relationship.

The Architecture of Disengagement Meets New Healthcare Spaces

Being inside a hospital can be illuminating if one pauses to appreciate it not only as a place where healthcare services are provided, but also as an urban space with stories to tell. As we walked around hospital campuses and on adjacent streets and sidewalks with neighborhood residents, we observed the way hospitals projected themselves to their communities. In Hartford and Aurora, among the most prominent structures facing communities were towering parking structures, which many residents saw as a sign that planners didn't concern themselves with how these facilities appeared to the communities looking at them from the outside. Making things worse, these structures were draped with prominent advertisements about the hospitals' rankings, which some residents found to be tone-deaf.

The developments described in chapter 3 include defensive strategies that dissuade locals from interacting with their institutions, and employees from engaging with their communities. Sometimes this defensive posture appears in architectural elements as well, such as large, featureless walls, obscured entryways, and tall fences limiting entry and access points. Barriers also come in the form of unwelcoming, dead spaces: moats of parking lots and battlements of garages. Hospitals offer spaces of opportunity and connection, but only if neighborhood residents find a way to overcome these obstacles.

The language residents use provides a window into how they perceive hospitals. A Cleveland organizer said the Clinic was "literally a neighborhood within a neighborhood. So, the Clinic neighborhood now resides within the actual Cleveland neighborhood. But there are just stark differences." Residents and hospital employees conjured a range of revealing language: interviewees in Hartford described the hospital as an "educational behemoth" and "large [and] intimidating," while those in Cleveland construed the Clinic as "a very sterile place, and imposing," and a "multinational behemoth." Clearly, these are not the words used to describe a place where community health is pursued. These perceptions are byproducts of inhospitable hospital design and planning. And while many of these individual decisions are the result of practical needs and decisions, the wider impression among locals is of facilities that have physically and symbolically turned their backs on their neighbors.

INVISIBLE FENCES AND PARKING LOTS

Respondents often discussed barriers. One interviewee, when describing Anschutz, explained: "The way I go, you're in residential areas and then: Boom! You cross Peoria [Street] and you're on the campus." Even when residents did not mention physical obstructions explicitly, they evoked them implicitly, via metaphor. One Hartford resident described a "kind of invisible wall" around the hospital, and another characterized it as a "fort." Similarly, a Cleveland resident mentioned "an invisible fence" around the University Circle. Recalling the history of the Clinic sending patients across town, another local characterized its main campus as a "referral citadel." Mario, an Auroran, remarked, "When you walk into a hospital, it's almost like you've walked into a separate dimension. You are in a world that is no longer your realm, but theirs . . ." In

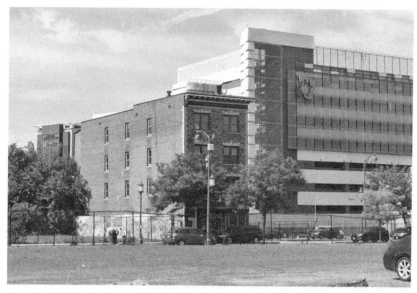

FIGURE 4.1. Parking lots, garages, and empty space around the periphery of Hartford Hospital (Photo by Wynn)

all three locations, residents referred to barriers in real and imagined ways. Considered together, these physical barriers comprise an "architecture of disengagement."

Certainly, hospitals have valid and understandable reasons to control access to their facilities. The safety of patients, employees, and even the public is at stake. Hospitals store sensitive health information and conduct delicate procedures. Perhaps most important for the purposes of this analysis, they follow protocols and procedures designed to limit the spread of infectious diseases, as required by the organizations tasked with accrediting and certifying the quality of their institutional practices.[12] Efficiency is also a factor leading to these spatial arrangements. Real estate agent Luis pointed to a hospital skywalk that allowed staff to move from building to building a few stories above street level. "I really feel," he said, "it would have been nice for the neighborhood kids and families to just walk around with the doctors, make them feel like they could walk the same road." Although the skywalk undoubtedly makes it easier for staff to move quickly without having to use elevators or pass through security checkpoints, for Luis, it symbolizes a "lack of connection."

Residents often point to parking as a symbol of disconnection. Residents can be quite understanding about hospitals' need to expand, but when once-beautiful homes or other establishments—such as the Hartford funeral home discussed in chapter 2—are replaced with parking lots instead of buildings that are more clearly worth the trade-off, communities feel disrespected. Residents were concerned that administrators saw their institutions as expendable targets for expansion, never thinking about how their communities might perceive these incursions or considering a more collaborative approach. Architecture also has implications for access. Tony Cherolis, a Hartford organizer who took an extended leave from the aerospace company Pratt and Whitney to work as a youth coordinator for the Center for Latino Progress, said Hartford Hospital's architecture was unwelcoming to the neighborhoods to its south, commenting, "They don't have an entrance on the street-facing side; it's in the parking lot . . . 40 percent of the households in these neighborhoods do not own a car."

When residents lose neighborhood resources for suburban patients' parking lots, the disdain can be understandable. Residents in all three locations were sensitive to the fact that boxy, unpleasant parking garages give the impression that their communities were being shown the "back end" of its medical campuses. Despite hospitals needing clear boundaries, the resulting architectural strategies produce a feeling of intimidation, exclusion, and disconnection.

COMMUNITY CLINICS

One of the chief contact points between communities and the healthcare system is the community clinic. Each of these hospitals have both on- and off-site clinics that serve as important spaces for contact, focused primarily, but not solely, on the provision of direct medical services.

Hartford Hospital Community Health, formerly the Brownstone Clinic, provides low-income, uninsured, and underinsured residents with mental health care, substance abuse treatment, basic dental care, HIV/AIDS treatment, primary care, and other services.[13] Every year, 40,000 patients visit the clinic, many of whom were referred by the ED, and most of whom have comorbidities and struggle to find housing. About half of the visits are for dental care, and Medicaid serves as the payment mechanism for 85 percent of these patients.[14] Pamela Clark, Nurse Manager at the Brownstone Clinic, described this care as "integral to the community at large and often undocumented or underinsured, noninsured, low-income [residents]." She told us the needs in the local community were significant, and explained that even if Brownstone could double its physical size, "We don't have enough providers . . . It's all based on the [medical school] residents and their rotations and when they can come here."

The DAWN Clinic is a student-run free clinic serving uninsured Aurorans. The website lists one of their goals as "serving the community surrounding the Anschutz Medical Campus," and notes that the clinic is "in the

heart of one of Colorado's most economically challenged and underserved regions," with "an uninsured rate upwards of 45 percent"[15] (see fig. 1.3 in chapter 1). Sallie Hanfelder, who was CEO of VA Eastern Colorado Health Care
System at the time of our interview, said the Anschutz entities have "wrapped
themselves into the community, especially the immigrant community," with
DAWN as a key piece of that effort.

The Cleveland Clinic opened the aforementioned Langston Hughes Community Health and Education Center in 2006. Sitting in the Fairfax neighborhood to the south of Hough and about one mile southwest of the main campus, the building is a renovated onetime branch library (see fig. 1.5). Shelly,
who worked in a local Community Development Corporation, recalled that
the Clinic selected the site based on the Black community's reverence for the
building. She concluded that, for the surrounding residents, the Center is "the
face of the Cleveland Clinic." It is accessible in more than one sense—it's easy
to arrive by foot and many of the staff members are locals. Shelly said that the
Center was more approachable as compared with the Clinic. According to Rachel, a Clinic administrator, the Center's "premise [was to] remove barriers."
Like the Hartford Hospital Community Health Clinic, this off-campus space
addresses specific community needs—in this case, primarily diabetes, hypertension, obesity, and HIV.

Off-site clinics and programs make sense. As Ellis in Aurora explained, "Creating off-site community-based clinics certainly makes it more accessible for
local residents to trust and come in and be seen." To varying degrees, having
clinics off-site also relieves demands for limited space on hospital campuses.
Administrators, however, touted neighborhood centers for helping residents
feel more comfortable than when visiting a larger, more impersonal hospital
complex.

Yet directing care to these facilities, even if they meet community needs,
raises a question about what kind of connectivity they engender. Do off-site
alternatives simply allow hospitals to avoid reworking their central facilities
and campuses and serve to further marginalize local communities, offering
what residents may perceive as separate-but-equal care? Further, if a facility
closes as commitments change, as happened with the Anschutz off-campus
site, where does that leave the local community?

OUTREACH AND "IN-REACH" PROGRAMS

A Cleveland Clinic administrator tasked with building relationships identified
the Clinic's goal as meeting the local communities "where they are at." Efforts

to achieve this goal include offering education programming on issues such as unhealthy diets, opioid addiction, and strokes, at venues such as schools, mobile van units, farmers markets, and health fairs.

These sites can be understood as temporary contact zones. We conducted an afternoon of alfresco interviews at one such site: a farmers market at Billings Forge, about a mile from the Hartford Hospital campus in Frog Hollow. The market, which is open year-round and is the largest of its kind in the city, provides access to healthy food for folks who live and work nearby. Insurance companies such as Aetna and The Hartford support the project by shuttling employees to the market to shop at the stalls and eat from the food trucks before being returned to work. If only in a small way, the shuttle service bridges the gap created by the Interstate-84 viaduct, which bisects the city (see fig. 1.6), and historically has limited investment in, and engagement with, the predominantly Latino and Hispanic communities. During the market's hours, the grassy area outside the historical brick and iron structures of Billings Forge becomes a vibrant, community-oriented space. To address food insecurity, the farmers market participates in a "Double Value Coupon Program," incentivizing customers to spend SNAP dollars on fresh produce and local goods.

There are also programs to bring the community on campus, serving as a kind of "in-reach." For example, Jefferson, a health researcher, said the Cleveland Clinic's Men's Minority Health Fair brings "thousands of people" to campus "for essentially free preventive [care] and identification for early risk factors." Another researcher, Angela, said the Clinic responded to community expectations by hosting summer programs for high school and college students, to help them "see what it's like to be a scientist, or a physician." Lara Ann Frey, who worked in program management and community navigation in the Denver area for years, touched on a similar point, commenting that job fairs on the Anschutz campus help people feel more comfortable applying for jobs. Physically, this navigation partnership has two locations: one on campus and another an eight-minute walk from campus, at the same library that once housed the Aurora Strong Resilience Center.[16] A former Anschutz employee who worked on some of these programs told us that they were intended to create a "non-intimidating" and "totally different atmosphere."

CAMPUS CAFETERIAS

Dining serves up another good example. One Hartfordite commented that they knew hospital employees who "worked there for 30 years and don't know there's a diner across the street." Our own experiences reinforced this assessment.

We ate several meals at Thai Farms, a restaurant directly across the street from Hartford Hospital, and despite its convenient location, it was usually almost empty during weekday lunch hours.

Francesca, the owner of a local Aurora restaurant just off campus, said she "got excited" when she learned of the new campus. She recalled that planners invited her to open a location in their food court, but when they said it would cost 30 percent of her earnings, she was shocked. She imagined that even in her original location, multitudes of workers and families would pass by her storefront. When the city required business owners in the area to comply with new zoning codes that required costly renovations, she invested in the improvements, planning on increased clientele. Once she reopened, however, she learned she wouldn't be allowed to advertise her business on campus, and the walk-in customers never materialized. "We were a lot better off before," she lamented. The long-standing neighborhood restaurant eventually closed.

Akin to a modern shopping mall or Vegas casino, the Anschutz campus boasts an impressive array of dining options to keep workers and patrons inside. Besides cafeterias, the campus offers fast food, Indian, Vietnamese Phở, Thai "street food," a brew pub, "handcrafted bagels," a Russian-themed coffee shop, and "Food Truck Wednesdays." In addition, new Panera, Chipotle, and Sonic franchises wreathe the campus, pulling customers from long-standing local restaurants with the draw of faster and cheaper food, according to Francesca. She believed Anschutz's food courts "killed" her business.

As with skywalks, campus cafeterias may make efficient sense on paper. Ed Tauer, who served as Aurora mayor for most of the time Anschutz was being planned, explained: "You can't walk for 25 minutes, have lunch, and walk 25 minutes back. You just took an hour and a half lunch to have a hamburger." But anchors have other options, of course. What if, for example, the Anschutz bus that shuttles employees from deep in the campus to the nearby light rail station made additional loops to neighborhood restaurants at lunchtime—just as Hartford's insurance companies take employees to the Billings Forge farmers market?[17] What if Francesca's invitation to the campus cafeteria was at a heavily subsidized rate? Adam Perkins, a city planner in the Denver area, claimed the hospital could have been better integrated into the neighborhood if they had opened their facades to Colfax Avenue, the major thoroughfare running along the campus's southern border. He called the choice not to do so a "missed opportunity." Clevelanders voiced similar complaints. As an urban planner explained, "When you look at [the Clinic's] buildings, you're seeing the backs of them. Then, they have all these courtyards [inside]. You can walk outside and you never have to look out onto the community." Similarly, one of Hartford's city planners said if she could change one thing, it would be to close the interior cafeterias in downtown anchor institutions. In her estimation—which harmonized with Francesca's experiences in Aurora—these cafeterias incentivize employees to stay on their campuses with "relatively cheap" and accessible food, and smaller establishments simply cannot compete. Closing the cafeterias, she said, would encourage people to "go spend money in the neighborhood and support street-level retail."

From satellite clinics to interior cafeterias, hospitals maintain barriers for practical reasons. For example, in all three locations, skywalks and tunnels ease access between buildings and insulate employees from inclement weather. These common connectors, however, also limit access to the surrounding communities, moving hospital personnel and patients around in a way that isolates life within the hospital from life directly outside on sidewalks and streets.

Where Changing Campus Roles Meet Communities of Color

Charles Rosenberg's *The Care of Strangers* highlights a curious moment wherein the history of hospitals created a new point of contact with patients. In 1874, patients were "still largely recruited from a culture very different from that which had socialized staff physicians and lay administrators," and thus Philadelphia's Pennsylvania Hospital hired an "officer of hygiene," whose job was to stop patients from using spittoons and emptying chamber pots in sinks and to keep patients' friends, relatives, and even dogs out of wards.[18] Rosenberg described how changes in the "social organization of the hospital" were made in the interest of managing the "enormous gap" between itself and its neighboring communities.

Hospitals are constantly changing, organizationally, in response to overlapping pressures and needs. In the contemporary era of community engagement, particularly with growing awareness of the communities of color that so often surround them, hospitals have made significant changes in their organizational structure to help them meet their neighboring communities. This section examines these organizational changes.

NAVIGATION AND TRANSLATION

As one marker of how hospitals prioritize roles that engage with communities, of the *U.S. News and World Report*'s list of top 50 hospitals in the U.S., we identified 37 clearly designated community engagement directors or specialists on staff.[19] These positions include, for example, Public Relations Associate (Mayo Clinic), Senior Community Outreach Specialist (Johns Hopkins), Community Relations Manager (University of Pennsylvania), and Director of

Community Benefit Systems and Planning (Cedars Sinai). The University of California–San Francisco has an entire organization dedicated to community interactions—the Center for Community Engagement. An administrator in one such post described their position as having "an internal- and an external-facing role." This administrator said their job included "developing relationships with community-based networks, including the networks with anchor institutions and community-based organizations but also economic development."[20] Administrative roles such as these are well positioned to join medical campus-based community-oriented working groups and campus offices.

There is, however, even greater growth in the number of healthcare professionals who, in the words of a nonprofit worker we interviewed, "bridge the gap between folks in the neighborhood and new [campus] services."[21] The purpose of these jobs is to connect patients to the various—though often fragmented—resources that American healthcare has on offer.

Unlike those in positions such as Vice President of Community Health, healthcare navigators and interpreters work on the frontlines of the hospital/community relationship. The staff in these roles serve as "critical liaisons" who orient patients to the different layers of care.[22] Although these staff provide a much-needed service, these positions have not always been instituted without advocacy from the community. Hartford's Hispanic Health Council (HHC) continues to work in this area, and early advocacy prompted the hospital to hire a "clerk-interpreter" who helps staff and patients communicate; the council was eventually awarded a grant from the Hartford Foundation for Public Giving for a full-time coordinator.

Other entities involved in the hospital/community relationship exist physically, organizationally, and symbolically outside the hospital while also being partially funded by it, like Hartford's Southside Institutions Neighborhood Alliance (SINA). Residents see SINA as a resource, but also understand that it serves as something of a buffer that defuses tensions arising in the hospital/community relationship. As a partnership across multiple institutions, SINA builds relationships across many organizations, but also exists outside the hospital's organizational structure, illustrating these organizations' need to partner while also working within the institutional cultures and structures of their partners.[23] Organizations such as SINA serve as stabilizing forces in a context in which some organizations have been around for decades but others seem to fold as quickly as they arise.

As noted in chapter 1, the 1964 Civil Rights Act requires that hospitals receiving federal funds provide "meaningful access" to patients. Such access necessitates greater cultural humility, and staffing of interpreters to improve outcomes and reduce errors.[24] Title VI of the Civil Rights Act prohibits discrimination based on race, color, or national origin; however, the legislation does not mandate federal or state funding for these positions or materials required to provide equal service.[25] Similarly, although Medicaid requires that hospitals receiving federal monies provide interpretation services, Medicaid does not require that states reimburse hospitals for those services.[26] The result of this complicated and incomplete policy landscape is a generally inadequate and certainly uneven approach to interpretation: families often serve as "ad hoc" interpreters (against federal law) or hospitals provide a patchwork of live interpreters and interpretation technologies.[27]

The history of organizational change in our sites was driven less by legal statute or the benevolence of the hospital and more by pragmatism—clinicians' basic need to communicate effectively with their patients—and local activism. For example, in response to the community mobilization mentioned in chapter 2, SINA hosted a Puerto Rican Forum, which served as the organizational birthplace of the Hispanic Health Council. SINA's inaugural director, Ivan Backer, said activists were, rightly, "very militant on translators."[28]

Although these staff provide a much-needed service, these positions have not always been instituted without advocacy from local residents. Hartford's Hispanic Health Council (HHC) continues to work in this area, and early advocacy prompted Hartford Hospital to hire a "clerk-interpreter" who helps staff and patients communicate; the council was eventually awarded a grant from the Hartford Foundation for Public Giving for a full-time coordinator. Hartford Hospital's lack of accessible interpretation services was the subject of a commentary published in the *Hartford Courant* in 2009; however, one Hartfordite, a Latina, reported that the hospital still doesn't have many interpreters, which has "left many feeling they're not treated respectfully."[29]

When we visited the HHC offices, located a block and a half from Hartford Hospital, we interviewed Grace Damio, Director of Research and Service Initiatives. She explained that HHC found that, even when there was a proficient Spanish speaker in a position at Hartford Hospital, the language differed so much across dialects that interpretation remained challenging. One caseworker gave the example of different variations of "ahorita/ahora," which might mean "now" to someone from Mexico and "later" to someone from Puerto Rico. When scheduling appointments or providing instructors for taking medicine at home, this distinction is critical.

When prompted, community leaders in Cleveland identified similar needs. Janey, a local nonprofit founder, noted that while the Clinic had made some progress, she felt equity remained an issue "across the board" in the city, and that there was a "lack of OB-GYNs and midwives of color." When asked about the progress, Shelly said most of the employees hired at the Clinic's Langston

Hughes Center were Black, "speak the same language" as residents, and were people whom residents "feel comfortable with." She continued, "They know their names when they come in and you don't have those types of relationships at the main campus of the Clinic." Other interviewees shared similar sentiments.

PATROLLING THE BORDER:
CAMPUS SECURITY AND COMMUNITY SAFETY

Mirroring the growth in new openings for interpreters and healthcare navigators, there has also been an expansion in hospital campus security operations. While this is not surprising considering the growth of medical campuses, here again, the unique role of health-centered anchor institutions in these areas tends to cast things in a slightly different light. Understanding hospital security is essential to understanding the hospital/neighborhood dynamic.[30]

Hospital websites contain ambiguous information about campus security, and for good reason: hospitals must balance the perception of their campuses as safe places and the perception that they have a reliable police force on campus. On the extreme side, Hartford Hospital's website has a true information deficit, providing almost no information available about campus security, save for several job opportunities and a feel-good story about a bomb-sniffing German shepherd named Nitro.

The "Visitor Information" section on Cleveland Clinic's website, however, contains a link to a "Police & Security" page, which promises 24/7 safety escorts and emergency response, safety awareness education, and of course, a series of emergency phone numbers.[31] The page also includes a tab on "Community Policing" with the following information: "In addition to its duties serving Cleveland Clinic patients, visitors and caregivers, our Police Department plays an active role in the community. It is our philosophy to be an active participant in community policing." At a later point, the page explicitly evokes commitments to "social responsibility and community involvement."

Because residents spoke about the Clinic's police force so often, we attempted to deepen our understanding of the organization. This proved to be a challenge. When we asked a Cleveland Clinic officer, Carl, about the size of the force, he replied that they "like to say we're about the third largest police department in Cuyahoga County." Carl, who was employed by the Clinic prior to the formation of the hospital police department, indicated that the Clinic had over 150 officers. A former Deputy Chief from the Cleveland Police Department headed the department. While 90 percent of U.S. police departments have fewer than 50 officers, the Clinic has over 150, University Hospitals has 80, and University Circle has about 25. Each of these units has formal agreements with surrounding departments to have full authority to enforce local, state, and even federal laws.

The Clinic's model is only one among many possible types, of course. University of Colorado Hospital, like many other hospitals, contracts with a billion-dollar corporation—Allied Universal Security Services, the third-largest contract security company in the U.S.—to provide security. The Anschutz campus employs 29 full-time law enforcement officers, some of whom have novel job titles such as "Security and Safety Ambassadors." Anschutz specifically notes that their officers are trained for de-escalation.[32]

Beyond the numbers, the work these campus security officers do, and where they do it, is notable. Perhaps the most surveilled spaces on hospital campuses are emergency departments,[33] which, as explained earlier, are key points of contact, an essential part of America's safety net, and places where society's most vulnerable arrive in times of crisis, especially in urban hospitals.[34] Security officers patrol other hospital spaces too. They might respond to opioid use in the hospital's public bathrooms or enter a patient's room via a "security standby request" made by staff—the rate of such requests is twice as high for Black patients as for white patients.[35] Perhaps more notably, campus police activity extends beyond the hospital walls, reaching into the surrounding streets, sidewalks, and lots. In cities, this presence can be robust. Overall, such activities deter neighbors from seeing hospitals as safe spaces, and therefore curb the desire to access needed care.[36]

Campus police forces attempt to balance the needs of the hospital and the needs of their communities. At times, these interests intersect in complex ways. As Carl, a Cleveland Clinic police officer, explained: "Well, the hospital is priority number one. Our caregivers, our student population, our docs, our nurses, are the priority. That's why we're here. However, the community part of it is also important. I like to say, if you have a safer Fairfax and safer Hough and safer Midtown, you'll have a safer main campus." When asked about the balance in their interactions with local residents, Carl estimated that their work was "60 percent community crime prevention and 40 percent community outreach."

One example of that 40 percent outreach was the Community Safety Awareness and Community Self Defense programs the Clinic police offered in partnership with the Cleveland Police Department in response to a rash of high-profile murders in the city. Commander Thomas McCartney said these programs were "about getting out into the community," and concluded that this work helps people feel comfortable giving an officer a call, but also put him in touch with neighborhood leaders. He continued: "I can't meet everybody, but I certainly meet the stakeholders. The residents are vital, but also the leaders or self-proclaimed leaders of the block groups and different organizations. It's key to policing. It is what policing is. It's not responding to lights and sirens." Other community outreach and awareness programs included "Coffee with a Cop" and attending safety fairs and block parties.

At times, however, the interests of campus safety and community needs clash. For example, an employee at the Aurora Resilience Center recalled an incident on the Anschutz campus that she believed reflected the campus-neighborhood relationship. Saying that security officers are "everywhere" on campus, she recalled how officers stopped and questioned a group from the neighborhood on their way to a resident leadership council meeting held on campus. According to what she heard, security officers were "thrown off by an interracial group on campus on a Saturday." She explained that the incident prompted the hospital to respond, including instructing security officers to shift toward "welcoming and helping [residents] find the building in case they get lost." Situations like this one alienate locals. More broadly, issues with campus safety and security raise significant concerns about bias and the treatment of the community.[37]

In Cleveland, as in Aurora, the campus's private police force moves into public spaces as well. Police at the Clinic even drive vehicles that closely resemble municipal police cruisers. Carl, a Clinic police officer, reported that the responsibilities of the campus police, in fact, overlap with those of the city police, per the formal agreement mentioned earlier. He explained: "There's been times where the Cleveland Police Department will call us to assist in a domestic [dispute] and say, 'Hey, can you all get there because we're tied up.' That is a continual thing that we do. But it's not unusual to see our police cars go at least a block or so away from the main campus." Community leaders and activists have criticized these off-campus excursions, calling the Clinic police their "Border Patrol" after a 2020 ProPublica report revealed that the force disproportionately charged and cited Black people.[38] An example from 2018 is notable: as two employees of a vendor that contracted with the Clinic jaywalked across Euclid Avenue in their work uniforms after finishing an eight-hour shift at the hospital's loading dock, a campus police officer detained them. One of the men sustained injuries from the encounter, necessitating a visit to the Clinic's own emergency department. In response to the report, the University Circle Police Chief offered a muted and curious response: "We are not looking at color, but basically trying to slow people down."[39]

A longtime Clevelander, Warren, described the Clinic's police force as "too aggressive" in their community outreach, and said it was staffed by "wannabe" cops. Another local wanted a *greater* "police presence," but one that was re-oriented: "I want the police like they used to be. When we knew them, they'd come by once in a while. Now it's only when there's a call that somebody's been shot, [or] maybe a domestic violence call . . . Just them being there would give a feeling of security for children. Code enforcement? Oh my god. If they would just go down my street, I would be so happy. Make these landlords enforce their property." Given campus police's status as an oft-armed private force with the authority to stop motorists and pedestrians to issue citations and make arrests, the line between crime prevention and community outreach tacks more toward the former, by all appearances.

Broadly, private police forces (including hospital security) operate with no or very little oversight. In 2018, the three private police forces in Cleveland's University Circle area agreed to establish civilian review boards within 30 days; however, only the Cleveland Clinic had done so at the time of the ProPublica report, two years later. Cleveland Municipal Court Judge Michael L. Nelson Sr. stated that, after establishing their original agreements with the city, these private police departments "never revisited" oversight and, instead, "set their own rules regardless of the consequences."[40]

For hospitals affiliated with a university, however, certain types of oversight and responsibilities come into play. The Jeanne Clery Disclosure of Campus Security Policy and Campus Crime Statistics Act—a 1990 federal statute requiring all colleges and universities receiving federal financial aid to collect and disclose crime data on and near their campuses—requires some hospitals to report on campus policing. For example, as part of the University of Colorado, the Anschutz campus must produce an annual Campus Security and Fire Report to maintain compliance.[41] The Clinic, as a private nonprofit, does not have to generate a report for its main campus operations, although some Clinic entities, such as the School of Diagnostic Imaging, are required to do so.[42] While all hospitals have reporting requirements for ED personnel concerning abuse, rape, gunshots, and other crimes, these requirements tend to be limited to their role as medical providers, and do not extend to their capacity as urban institutions.

In hospitals that fall under the Clery Act, the zones of interaction between hospitals and communities tend to be better defined. Clery defines "on campus" as properties owned or occupied by a university or college *and* non-campus spaces, including public property, along borders and internal to a campus that is used to support the institution.[43] As explained in detail in chapter 6, something like a Clery Act for hospitals could help secure their role as community anchors.

ON CULTURAL HUMILITY

When considering new hospital roles and campus entities, there is a need for greater awareness and knowledge, both inside and outside hospital walls. In the past, this pursuit of openness, empathy, and commitment to understand the backgrounds of patients has been described in medical spaces as cultural competence, or more recently, cultural humility. The latter term emphasizes the futility in trying to learn every cultural custom or even language one might encounter as a healthcare professional. The limitation of this approach, however, lies in its focus on individual interactions between healthcare professionals and patients. As we introduced in chapter 1, we now know that healthcare services are not nearly as consequential as the broader social environments in shaping health. Jonathan Metzl, a well-known psychiatrist and sociologist, coined the term *structural competence*, to emphasize a new type of knowledge that is needed in medicine. Structural competence implies understanding the scope of health disparities affecting both patients and communities, particularly those who are stigmatized or marginalized, and recognizing the structural factors that underlie the health of populations.[44] Indeed, in our interviews, themes of racism, ethnocentrism, and language arose repeatedly, echoing research that shows how a lack of structural competence strains relationships between hospitals and communities.[45]

Sherrie, a white medical professional in Cleveland, made the connection between the deep memories of communities (discussed in chapter 2) and the organizational shifts discussed above. She said that the Community Advisory Board was a space for patients to confide in her, discuss a lack of trust in the hospital, and help her understand that "we have this legacy in healthcare, of experimenting on slaves, experimenting on Black people, without consent." She continued by acknowledging that she "has to own that and grapple with it, to understand how that affects our patients today." These conversations contextualize her patients' decisions, for example, not to vaccinate their children; however, they also shape plans for a new Center for Women and Children. Sherrie said the issue is as much about her educating herself as a clinician as it is "for us as an institution." Spaces such as the Community Advisory Board provided opportunities to build trust, but she knew these efforts wouldn't be successful without "naming and talking about systemic racism."

Kenneth, who works in community engagement in Cleveland, also addressed the role of race in the hospital/community relationship. He characterized healthcare institutions as taking a "trickle-down" approach to addressing racism, asking senior-level executives to take part in training on racism, and hoping their participation would "encourage others who are on the ground or mid-level execs to do it as well."[46] Community advisory boards, which exist in many municipalities, are spaces where the pressure to address racism can "percolate up." Kenneth described how the Community Health Action Team (CHAT), which is composed of healthcare professionals and residents, identified specific policies and practices that perpetuate healthcare inequalities. Participants, for example, pointed out that urban patients pay for parking while suburban hospitals offer free parking.

These are examples of perhaps the most important theme that emerged with respect to the contact zones where the personnel associated with organizational changes in healthcare (e.g., interpreters and campus safety officers) interact with the surrounding neighborhoods, which tend to be communities of color. While scholars have found that discussions about cultural competency in healthcare were limited in the early 2000s, the idea wasn't entirely foreign to the hospital administrators we interviewed.[47] Still, as Cleveland's Heidi Gartland explained, administrators have to catch up: "We don't have the cultural competency; we don't understand trust and mistrust, and racial bias as it relates to a structural bias." She said the institution has to go through a "full odyssey," but that the journey ahead "isn't entirely ours." Despite recognizing the need for hospitals to fund these efforts, Gartland concluded that this road needs to be traveled in partnership with neighboring communities.

Working in the Zone: Actors and Organizations
Operating amid Barriers

Foundations played key roles in all three research sites, offering grants for arts, education, and youth programs, but also bringing together city entities to achieve community-oriented goals. For example, when issues of campus policing arose, former University Circle Inc. president Chris Ronayne asked the Cleveland Foundation, an influential community nonprofit, to bring together the private and public police agencies of the University Circle to discuss how they patrol the hospital and its surroundings. According to the ProPublica report, Ronayne said, "I think this is an opportunity to change tack on a systemic problem," adding: "One department can't do it alone."

The Cleveland Foundation—the world's first community foundation with $2.5 billion in assets—was at the center of the relationship between the University Circle hospitals and their neighborhoods. As mentioned in chapter 1, the Foundation established GUCI in 2005 and funded the European trip for GUCI officials and lawmakers to learn about worker-owned cooperatives as they worked to launch the Evergreen Cooperatives. The Denver Foundation played a similar convening role in getting the University of Colorado Hospital to reorient its mission and develop local hiring and living programs, drawing on lessons learned from Cleveland. In 1969, a small Hartford Foundation grant was used to hire a community relations officer for Trinity College and Frog Hollow—a position that expanded into the SINA organization.

Over the last few decades, anchor institutions warmed to the idea of nearby community-based organizations having a greater say in their affairs.[48] The pace of this change and the reasons underlying it depend on the specific ecology of relationships. Myriad community-based organizations (CBOs) and city officials work in the spaces between hospitals and communities, but every urban neighborhood has different amounts of organizational resources, and not all of these embedded organizations have the same capacity.[49] Sometimes the work of these intermediary groups and individuals benefits residents, while other times their efforts falter, placing relationships at risk and provoking local frustrations.

The discussions above have already flagged many actors and organizations who engage "in the in-between" social spaces. We encountered leaders of a multitude of community organizations: nonprofits, CBOs, community development corporations and community development financial institutions, tech incubators, foundations, community connectors, federally qualified health centers (FQHCs), campus police, city government, and local businesses. Further, as noted above, hospitals also attempt to bridge some of the large social, cultural, and geographic gaps between their organizations and their communities via important organizational positions.

Social scientists, depending on their methodological orientation, might call these actors and organizations "brokers," "intermediaries," or "boundary spanners."[50] In many of the interviews, residents and hospital personnel used the terms "change agents" or "conveners." The brokerage work occurring at the individual and organizational levels in healthcare takes many forms.[51] Institutions such as childcare facilities, churches, recreation centers, and community-based organizations broker vital resources for vulnerable neighbors while also responding to a variety of threats. Further, pivotal individuals, whether nurses or emergency medical technicians, can wield their social capital to unite community groups and these institutions.[52]

Some of these entities exist within the operating budgets of the hospitals (e.g., vice presidents and campus police), while others exist with little-to-no financial connection to the hospital. Many, however, are partially funded by the hospitals, have some ties with them (e.g., hospital employees are board members), or aspire to have such connections. Thus, these embedded institutions can be independent (mostly financially independent of healthcare centers), dependent (strong financial ties with healthcare organizations), or exogenous (existing outside the field of healthcare yet playing a role in communities). Independent organizations can include local churches or businesses that do not contract with the hospitals but fill important roles within communities and often serve as a bridge between the hospital and their communities. Dependent organizations can range from those receiving large financial contributions (e.g., GUCI, SINA) to those operating on thinner margins and receiving occasional contributions from anchors. Exogenous organizations and actors include city, county, and state health departments and former politicians; however, few major players in these ecosystems are totally outside a hospital's reach.[53]

Melvyn Colón, the Executive Director of SINA, characterized the organization as a "convener." When asked how SINA conducts its work, he explained that the group first hosts stakeholders, policymakers, philanthropic groups, and city government officials to "generate discussion and to get other people's insights and ideas" and marshal some "force" behind the brainstorming. SINA then holds a second meeting for "community residents and nonprofit partners" to communicate what resources and options are available to the neighborhood residents.

While CBOs existed for decades prior, the 1964 Economic Opportunity Act included a "Special Impact Program" that created a new 501(c)(3) nonprofit: community development corporations, or CDCs.[54] The number of CDCs has grown from 2,000 in 1995 to over 8,000 today.[55] Fairfax Renaissance Development Corporation, one of the Clinic's major partners, is one of them. Courtney, a community organizer in the city, said, "We have a unique CDC system here, where each neighborhood has its anchor CDC that is the gatekeeper for a lot of things going on." CDCs also serve as intermediaries, as unelected yet "authorized representatives of the city's neighborhoods, empowered with quasi-governmental responsibilities and a strong bent toward economic growth."[56] While Kristen Morris at the Cleveland Clinic noted that the city is "moving away" from the model, CDCs continue to shape community politics in Cleveland.

BREAKING BARRIERS AMID COMPETING AGENDAS

Examples from two key actors who worked with hospitals and communities— a Hartford city official who operated separately from the hospital and the community, and a key administrator who worked from within the Cleveland Clinic—illustrate how individuals can change contact zones "on the ground."

First, Ron Pepin, the planner for the City of Hartford who has worked in

Hartford's Office of Small Business and Community Development, spoke about his struggles with the city's anchor institutions. His office was often engaged in efforts to nudge anchor institutions to design buildings that "fit" with the neighborhood, and to be "more open, more integrated, more connected to the community." He lamented, however, that he "frequently lost those battles."

Ron described the placement of a doorway to illustrate how city oversight and compromise shape a contact point that we could characterize as the "architecture of disengagement." After agreeing to the city's request to preserve a building rather than tear it down, Hartford Hospital wanted the front entrance to be "decorative" and to place the building's only access point in the back, facing a secluded parking lot. Ron recounted, "We were like, 'Well, no. We want you to have a permeable entrance on the street. If someone's looking for the entrance, they should be able to walk right off the sidewalk into your building.'" This kind of back-and-forth, aided by the city's power in land-use controls, led to compromise. City leaders from all three sites sometimes characterized these kinds of negotiations with hospitals as difficult, using terms such as "conflictual," "tough sledding," and "contentious." Ron called these negotiations an "interesting dance," adding: "You love them [anchors] because they're great employers . . . They give living-wage jobs, and they're growing like mad. The other side of it is we also believe they could make a neighborhood really vibrant. Their campus should extend to the surrounding neighborhood."

Alex, an employee at the Cleveland Clinic, offered another example of how individuals influence contact zones. He explained, "When we do things internally, we take that to the community to see how the community will receive it because we do nothing in a vacuum. We may have great ideas, but we want to get the community's feedback. I have an advisory panel I meet with quarterly, and we talk about projects that we're working on, opportunities we're getting ready to go out to bid on in the next 6–12 months out, and we really get them to help us in our effort." Alex understood the Clinic's procurement power as offering a great deal of leverage to alter relationships between the hospital and local communities.

Beyond Ron Pepin and Alex, there are many people and organizations working with hospitals, often with competing agendas. In these communities, organizational brokers work to attain meaningful results. In Hartford, the Hispanic Health Council successfully developed cultural humility among local healthcare providers, although, according to Grace Damio, demand outstrips capacity. Cleveland CBOs such as Neighborhood Progress and the Racial Equity Institute hold training sessions for healthcare workers. Max, a Cleveland nonprofit worker, noted that these trainings and workshops "amplify the voice of people in the Black community" and "lead conversations on race." And Zoe, a high-level administrator at the Cleveland Clinic, said her organization works with these local groups to publicize opportunities, offer job interview coaching, and conduct recruitment.

This kind of brokering can be a tense process. Hospitals and communities do not possess similar levels of resources, a point most hospital administrators acknowledged. One administrator, for example, commented that the Clinic had to walk a "weird kind of line" as both a partner that many smaller organizations link with but also an institution that holds the capacity to "change markets." She continued: "We then would ask our partners—they could be a Boys and Girls Club, an art and cultural institution, a school, a church— that they use our resources, whether it's capital or money, to focus in geographic areas where we can see the greatest impact. . . . Folks look to us, but at the same time we have to sort of tamp it down just a little so that we can be a true partner and not sort of drive everything." This awareness of the hospitals' disproportionate power was refreshing and commendable. The healthcare industry, however, has been discussing cultural competency for decades without effectuating much change in our cases. Many interviewees, both inside and outside the three hospitals, believed that this kind of sensitivity, particularly in thinking about hiring multilingual workers, remains a major unfulfilled goal.

Joel Cruz, a former City Councilor and the Director of Hartford's Institute for the Hispanic Family, said his community-based nonprofit offers a variety of health-related services to children and seniors. The organization hosts pediatricians and nutritionists from Connecticut Children's who present programs on obesity and cooking. In addition, a mobile health van from Charter Oak Health Center (an FQHC) arrives once a week to offer routine checkups and free blood pressure tests. Remarkably, Cruz's organization was not at the far edge of the city but *directly across the street from Hartford Hospital.* Cruz's insistence that this was an important location for such work was a stark reminder of the paradox of medically underserved communities existing in the shadow of elite healthcare institutions.

CDCs are influenced by complex dynamics. As Anita, a Cleveland city planner, explained, CDCs themselves often have contested agendas. Important dynamics are at play in Cleveland's CDC landscape. First, a series of norms generally unite the city's CDCs, but each organization has its own, slightly different mission.[57] For example, some focus on residency-based assistance while others focus on economic development. According to Courtney, some CDCs "organize many events . . . health fairs, safety fairs, back-to-school fairs, and so

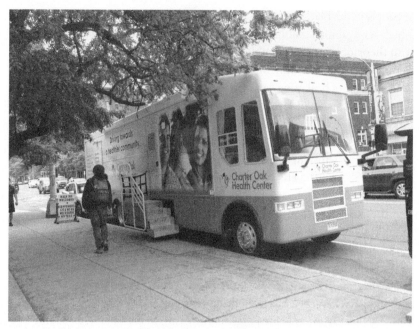

FIGURE 4.2. A Charter Oak Health (FQHC) mobile van parked at the Hartford Public Library; a Hartford Hospital banner is visible in the background (Photo by Wynn)

on," and cater to the specific dynamics of their neighborhoods. Second, CDCs tend to be heavily influenced by their respective city councilors who, according to Lee Lazar, "[set] aside money for them." Third, as Chris Stocking noted, there is often a "disconnect" between the CDC and the neighboring communities, because CDCs "play more of a role in developing neighborhoods for businesses, which might not be the type of development that residents would like to see." For this reason, residents sometimes criticized CDCs (and CBOs), perceiving them as pawns for the elite institutions they partner with. Politicians, corporations, and nonprofit anchor institutions like these hospitals frequently flaunt their "engagement with the community" by highlighting their work with these organizations.

A bird's-eye view of these interactions in Cleveland reveals that the Clinic and other GUCI institutions lean toward working with Fairfax's CDC over Hough's. Anita said this preference is the reason Fairfax has a "relatively comfortable relationship with the Clinic and the expansion that they're doing; they're cooperating." She remarked that the Clinic used the Fairfax CDC as their "front to get the things that they want." Clearly, then, a neighborhood's CDC (or lack of a functioning one) informs how communities and hospitals interact.

KEY PERSONNEL AND STAFFING
FROM THE COMMUNITY

Prior research shows that if stakeholders view brokers as legitimate and engage with partners frequently, intergroup relationships can improve.[58] In conversations with people on all sides of these relationships, however, interviewees placed a great deal of value on not just the initiatives these actors and organizations implement, but also who is making contact in the contact zone.

Elizabeth, a Hartford resident who worked in addiction services, emphasized the importance of hiring the right person in these intermediary roles. It is not enough, she concluded, to have a "community connector" healthcare professional presenting to a community group whose members are Black. She continued, "You need to have a person who's culturally competent . . . to make the presentation, form the relationship, establish the rapport, and it shouldn't matter what racial group the person is." Similarly, Colón said SINA was planning to hire a career navigator, which they have since done—the organization hired an experienced employment professional with expertise in career counseling for and coaching of dislocated workers.

Given these conversations, it is unsurprising but commendable that hospitals are hiring from their local communities, and local community groups aim to have former and current hospital administrators serve in their organizations. The Cleveland Clinic has hired people who worked with and even led local CDCs. Keith, Director of Cleveland's Health-Tech Corridor, noted how important it was that the Clinic recruited residents with strong ties within the community, saying this practice lends respect and credibility to any initiative. And, in like fashion, while a CBO such as the Hispanic Health Council might have a bristly relationship with Hartford Hospital, they also have hospital administrators as occasional board members, and partner with the hospital in outreach efforts, for example, a recent COVID-19 vaccine clinic.

These examples show that it's not just that these organizations staff community-facing positions, but that they staff them with people who have sufficient cultural sensitivity and are committed to this work. Healthcare navigators and interpreters are crucial for residents to gain access to hospital services. Organizations know there are many gaps that must be bridged—including divides in language, terminology, culture, history, and perhaps goals—when connecting the local hospitals with surrounding communities.

Different intermediaries are, as expected, differently positioned. Some are vice presidents and others are board members of community groups; some are organizations with deep pockets and others are nonprofits with meager financial resources. As a result, these intermediaries hold different visions and aims, as well as varying levels of trust and connectivity with others. Clearly, however, the importance of and growth in the norms of community involvement and collaboration have shown that these brokers and intermediaries must work across traditional boundaries, even when it is difficult to do so. How and to what extent these actors are able to accomplish this, of course, is part of the story of changes in institutional culture captured in this book.

Conclusion: The Fence and Ambulance

Physicians' offices sometimes feature an abbreviated version of "The Ambulance Down in the Valley," an old poem by Joseph Malins, on their waiting-room walls. (Singer-songwriter John Denver did a version of this for his concert tours.) Kevin, a professor near one of the three research sites, described the poem as a rumination about where to target healthcare initiatives—whether to place a fence at the top of a hill (as a preventive measure) or place an ambulance down in the valley (to help those who fall and injure themselves). Kevin said: "I think hospitals have seen themselves as the ambulance at the bottom of the hill. And yet they have been beneficiaries of the same forces of racism that the privileged elite [wield] against people in the community." The poem states the problem plainly enough: Where is the point of contact for healthcare? In prevention or in acute care?

This chapter reorients these questions around the idea of contact zones, but also demonstrates that a wide range of new actors and institutions move in often dynamic ways within these spaces. From the growth of high-level administration positions to increases in the number of ground-level healthcare interpreters, from community/hospital groups such as Community Health Action Team (CHAT) and campus-community partnerships such as SINA to more specific entities such as the Cleveland Clinic's supplier diversity council, such institutional change has been a long time coming.

While the details differ across sites, scholars and activists have made broad normative arguments for why hospitals must expand opportunities—more contact, more physical places—to connect with their communities. We have attempted to dislodge the traditional notion of emergency departments and exam rooms as the primary points of access, and to invite greater innovation by identifying spaces that host significant encounters between institution and neighborhood; naming the barriers, limitations, and opportunities in these spaces; and identifying the key players at these sites.

The good news is that some of the hospital administrators we interviewed discussed how hospital spaces can and should play a role in their communities. Michael Modic, a former physician at the Cleveland Clinic, offered a broad vision: "One of the things I think is critical is that the healthcare facility is primarily devoted to being a resource to the community [and should] have a point for communion, whether it's [an] education environment, whether it's conferencing, whether it's a civic, whether it's a social center, whatever it is." Deborah, a local grants officer, also focused on points of contact between the hospital and local communities, noting that while there has long been an "invisible wall" around the Clinic, GUCI has made efforts to "really break down those walls [and] create more entry points, two-way entry points, for the residents to the hospitals, and hospitals into the neighborhoods."

Rethinking a hospital's interactions with its neighboring communities requires taking a perspective that incorporates physical, social, and symbolic spaces and, importantly, how they intersect with health and socioeconomic inequalities. Hospitals must wrestle with the inequalities that are part of a municipality's history and those that are part of the community members' experiences with healthcare and medicine—both of which are, at least in part, economic in nature. A sensitivity to the factors that influence these physical, social, and symbolic spaces can lead to a nuanced understanding of the hospital/community relationship.

5

Ambiguous Obligations and Mixed Expectations

We really try to make sure that no matter where the Cleveland Clinic is, there is a certain expectation of what it's like as a neighbor.

KRISTEN MORRIS, former Chief Government and Community Relations Officer, Cleveland Clinic

The relationship between hospitals and communities is clearly complex, but a key question underlying this relationship is straightforward: What can communities expect from their hospitals? Interviewees, both inside and outside our hospitals, talked about a wide range of things hospitals *can* and *should* do. These expectations were based on different underlying assumptions, perspectives, and institutional and other positional contexts.

Many residents can imagine how their own experiences would differ from those of well-heeled VIP patients—indeed, guided tours and informal conversations with hospital personnel often highlighted the excellent care given to A-list patients. While some residents might expect no more from hospitals than simply upholding their fundamental Hippocratic values—"First, do no harm"—some community members said they did expect more from the large medical institutions in their neighborhoods. Some expected their hospitals to improve their lives, and the lives of nearby residents.

University Circle nonprofit worker Kevin, whose quote about the ambulance at the bottom of the hill was at the end of the previous chapter, continued those thoughts by saying: "I can envision a day when a hospital is about creating value for people in the community . . . things that they need that might help connect them to the social determinants of health . . . income, education, healthy environment, recreation, a sense of purpose, all of those things that a lot of which have been taken away from communities by the forces of racism essentially." These expectations represent community members' hopes that hospitals will shift their efforts and resources upstream toward prevention; they echo the desire expressed by other respondents for an approach that transcends biomedical models and "downstream" clinical healthcare services. Neighbors are hoping for a fence, not an ambulance.

Coming up against these expectations are the hospitals, with their thoughtfully crafted mission and values statements emblazoned on web pages, billboards, and television ads. Anschutz Medical Center commercials trumpet their work as "a calling." A Hartford Hospital Bone and Joint Institute commercial tells viewers their surgeons "rock." Despite these cheerful claims, which may sometimes ring hollow for residents, hospital administrators know their institutions have a long way to go to satisfy their neighbors. For administrators such as Kristen Morris, whose quote opens the chapter, expectations are significant parts of a hospital's identity. The work isn't easy. As the passive language of Morris's formulation suggests, expectation-setting is a massive multi-player collective project in which powerful anchors can be more or less influential. Further, despite the asymmetry of power between hospitals and their communities, locals have some ability to poke and prod these neighborhood heavyweights, sometimes through the media and political action.

Residents, local and federal governmental agents, and other actors are increasingly interested in how hospitals are—or are not—meeting the public's expectations, and therefore are raising new questions: Are billing practices fair? What should communities expect a hospital or medical center to do about interpersonal and structural racism? What should these institutions do about poor housing stock, crime, food deserts, and persistent income and wealth inequality?

Building on the previous chapters, this chapter outlines the factors that inform these expectations to create a more nuanced understanding of this landscape of obligations and promises. To set the stage for the final chapter, which puts forth policy recommendations for improving population health through hospital/community relationships, this penultimate chapter explores how formal and informal expectations coalesce.

What Informs Expectations?

Though there can be reasonable disagreement about what a hospital should or can do for the surrounding communities, expectations generally cohere around familiar themes. The interviews point to four broad categories that shed light on the collective negotiation of expectations both inside and outside hospitals: 1) trust in medical institutions, 2) formal-legal obligations, 3) hospital mission, and 4) perceived capacity.

Residents weren't always certain about these expectations, but their concerns centered around ensuring their communities' basic needs were met. Folks who work in these hospitals often have expectations too. As we discuss below, hospital workers sometimes view managing expectations as just as important as meeting them.

TRUST AND CONFIDENCE IN MEDICAL INSTITUTIONS

Political scientist Francis Fukuyama argued that trust in institutions is an important part of how people form expectations.[1] Overall, Americans have varying levels of trust in institutions, professionals, and leaders. Trust in the medical system, for example, differs from trust in other social institutions. The best social science data we have on the question is generally framed in terms of "confidence" in institutions, which serves as a decent proxy for trust. As table 5.1 shows, in recent years different institutions have received varying degrees of public confidence.

The data in table 5.1 show that confidence in the medical system rose sharply between 2019 and 2020 (when it was third highest, behind "the military" and "small business"), but then experienced the second-largest loss of confidence during the ensuing months of the pandemic, dropping below "the police." It's unclear, however, if the earlier rise in confidence in medicine is attributable to general positive feelings in the early months of the COVID-19 pandemic.

Many Americans adopt an at least nominally anti-government position, undercutting the potentially positive role of local, state, and federal policies supporting improved healthcare and oversight of these institutions.[2] This distrust in government boiled over during the 2020 presidential campaign and

TABLE 5.1. Confidence in institutions, 2019–2021 (percent who have "a great deal" or "quite a lot" of confidence)

	2019	2020	2021	% Change 2020–2021
Public schools	29	41	32	−9
The medical system	36	51	44	−7
Small business	68	75	70	−5
The church or organized religion	36	42	37	−5
Banks	30	38	33	−5
The U.S. Supreme Court	38	40	36	−4
The criminal justice system	24	24	20	−4
The military	73	72	69	−3
Technology companies	—	32	29	−3
Organized labor	29	31	28	−3
Newspapers	23	24	21	−3
Television news	18	18	16	−2
The presidency	38	39	38	−1
Big business	23	19	18	−1
Congress	11	13	12	−1
The police	53	48	51	3

Source: https://news.gallup.com/poll/352316/americans-confidence-major-institutions-dips.aspx.

election, when it was compounded by a sense that government and other institutions had failed, on various levels, to respond effectively to the COVID-19
pandemic.[3] Political scientist Suzanne Mettler has argued that many Americans believe the solutions to public problems should be either individualized
or privatized, while the governmental systems underpinning U.S. life remain
hidden or "submerged," meaning the average American cannot appreciate the
extent of the government's role, especially in promoting safety and health.[4]

Though residents rarely voiced anti-government sentiments, some municipal leaders said this thinking was common. For example, when Anschutz was
becoming a reality, Ed Tauer was mayor of Aurora. Ed offered a sense of the
community's position at the time, especially their expectations of the government's role in improving community health: "Oh, God, no. Nobody trusts you.
You're the government. Are you serious? Nobody trusts us." Tauer's perspective is important when considering the important role the government played
in orchestrating the Anschutz project, overseeing the conversion of a military
base—the epitome of a government facility—into a medical campus. The medical center's status as a public hospital complicates this critique of the government; the facilities on the Anschutz Medical Campus are government—that
is, public—entities instead of private nonprofits. Tauer recounted that to navigate this lack of trust, the city partnered with community groups to create
community-centered programming and then worked with local leaders to
"get the word out." He continued: "[We were] saying, 'Help us reach these people so that they know that this is what we're going to do,' and going out to the
community and saying, 'All right, everyone's going to be concerned that we're
just running over people. We're not. Let us show you what we're doing.' By
the time you get done showing them, they go, 'Okay, you're actually making a
real effort.'" Yet when considered carefully, Tauer's skepticism about the role
of government in hospital/community collaborations complements the idea
that, under the right conditions, government can play a generative role.[5]

FORMAL-LEGAL OBLIGATIONS

We spoke with some hospital neighbors who expected very little from their hospitals and others who believed hospitals did enough. Residents' expectations
of hospitals and hospitals' expectations of themselves stem from a diffuse sense
of formal responsibility. As outlined in chapter 1, Community Health Needs
Assessments mandated by the Affordable Care Act, as well as other community benefit obligations triggered by federal tax-exemption status, compel hospitals to both gauge and address community needs. There is, however, disagreement and misunderstanding about the technical aspects of community

benefit obligations, and hospitals vary dramatically in terms of their under-standing of the scope and sufficiency of the work they do.[6]

Research shows that higher levels of education and cultural awareness are associated with increased expectations regarding legal responsibility.[7] Certainly, locals in our three cities expressed a range of views on the legal obligations of community benefit. Aurora resident Valeria, for example, believed it was the hospital's "duty to give back as much as they can," though she didn't define the scope or specific aims of this expectation of "giving back." In many ways, Vale-ria's response was typical; many residents (understandably) mentioned "duty" or "obligation" without referencing legal or other formal requirements.

Respondents who were more closely connected to local organizations, un-surprisingly, had greater expectations. Nonprofit workers in community orga-nizations relevant to hospitals were acutely aware that hospitals had a certain level of responsibility to their communities. For example, Jenny, who worked at a Cleveland community-planning CBO, described her expectations for the Clinic as follows: "I think any . . . nonprofit has an obligation to do good in the community while meeting their expectations as a healthcare provider and employer. Their obligations are obviously, first, to their patients, and sec-ond, to their staff, but their community has to be hugely important because when you look at the rate of infant mortality next to the Cleveland Clinic, it's heartbreaking when you realize [there is] world-class healthcare three blocks north of these poor mothers." While Valeria and Jenny were both cognizant of the nonprofit status of their hospitals and the expectation of providing di-rect services to residents, and Jenny could articulate the obligations grounded in that status in detail, very few residents knew their local hospitals were obli-gated to sponsor nonmedical and other outreach programs. Legal obligations can only set expectations if people are aware of them.

Within the broader medical profession there is a sense that hospitals are doing enough or even more than enough, a sentiment shared by some locals. A recent industry-sponsored report commissioned by the American Hospital Association, for example, claimed that U.S. nonprofit hospitals' community work "far exceed[s]" the tax benefits they receive.[8] Researchers and policy-makers remain less convinced, however, noting, for example, the "fair-share deficits" we outline in chapter 1.

As anticipated, hospital administrators were keenly aware of these expec-tations and took them seriously in the interviews; after all, compliance can be a high-stakes consideration for these institutions. Some aspects of the lack of clarity that exists about the scope of IRS requirements are the result of a pur-poseful underspecification of policy on the part of Congress, intended to af-ford hospitals flexibility.[9]

Most administrators recognized the ambiguous nature of these requirements. When they spoke about the hospital's community work, they did not want to imply that their good deeds were mere compliance, rather than the satisfaction of altruistic or moral aims. Mary Stuart, Director of Health Equity at St. Francis Hospital in Hartford, acknowledged that hospitals have "tremendous" resources outside of clinical care and that community-oriented work holds a lower priority: "We're a clinical organization. We should be good at that, and we should make sure we've got that down. I think that, because we're a large institution with lots of different resources and skill sets that are outside of the clinical setting, we need to organize ourselves to leverage that for the community as well." Hospital leaders like Mary, embedded in the changing healthcare landscape, often expect more from their institutions.

HOSPITAL MISSION

Administrators emphasized their institutions' missions rather than compliance with formal-legal requirements. Both residents and administrators described institutional missions in ambiguous ways, simultaneously intentional and clear but also vague and subjective. As key aspects of public relations, mission statements are also a piece of the expectations puzzle.

Institutions often define their missions in qualitatively different ways. "Eds and Meds" are distinct from large corporations and other anchor institutions in that the specific nature of their work—education and health—entails high-minded expectations of benevolence and care. It is unclear whether residents recognize the formal definitions of these missions *vis-à-vis* communities. In understanding hospitals' missions, however, it is useful to look past formal statements, which are more like platitudes with little to say about the actual mission (see table 5.2).[10]

Their vacuousness notwithstanding, these statements signal how hospitals want to be seen by employees, patients, and the wider public. For example, both the Cleveland Clinic and Hartford Hospital include geographic ambitions in their vision statements, with the Clinic hoping to become "the best place for care anywhere" and Hartford Hospital promoting its ambition to cultivate a wider national reputation. All three mission statements identify individuals of various sorts ("lives/life," "people") as their focus. These statements, as expected, deploy the word "care," though only to evoke direct medical services, as opposed to, for example, population health. The Anschutz mission statement is somewhat more expansive in its mention of "improving lives," and a generous reader could interpret that as including communities, but only Hartford Hospital's statement explicitly mentions community. Notably, the Cleveland

TABLE 5.2. Hospital mission statements

Institution	Mission statement	Vision statement
Anschutz Medical Center (CU Health)	"We improve lives. In big ways through learning, healing, and discovery. In small, personal ways through human connection. But in all ways, we improve lives."	"From health care to health."
Cleveland Clinic	"Caring for life, researching for health, educating those who serve."	"To be the best place for care anywhere and the best place to work in healthcare."
Hartford Hospital	"To improve the health and healing of the people and communities we serve."	"To be nationally respected for excellence in patient care and most trusted for personalized coordinated care."

Sources: https://my.clevelandclinic.org/about/overview/who-we-are/mission-vision-values; https://hartford hospital.org/about-hh/mission-vision-values; https://www.uchealth.org/about/.

Clinic refers to its internal workplace as a point of focus, suggesting an inward rather than outward perspective. It is precisely the space *between* this inward and outward focus, of course, that is being negotiated within the broader question of expectations.

Hospital neighbors had understandably less refined ideas about the hospitals' missions. When we asked nonprofit worker Claudia for her thoughts on the Clinic's mission, she reported that while she was relieved to have a prestigious hospital nearby, she was unsure of its mission: "I think they're doing a great job for what they are, but in terms of community responsibility . . . I don't know," she said, pausing before continuing, "I don't know their guiding principles . . . above the medical piece." Other residents had similar difficulties defining missions. When pondering the role of the Clinic in the Hough community and whether it should extend beyond medicine, Mansfield Frazier concluded: "They're not in the business of making widgets. They're in the business of promoting health." An Auroran described the matter in blunter terms: "Their approach is 'Money, money, money,' and that's it."

From the community's perspective, mission statements do not clarify hospitals' roles as teaching institutions with sometimes expansive, and well-funded, research operations. In traditional terms, teaching and research in healthcare are often seen as inward-facing activities, focused on medicine itself, with a secondary commitment to maintaining and improving the larger healthcare system through workforce training and new forms of biomedical knowledge. Just how biomedical research and teaching can benefit the communities outside a hospital raises broader questions about who benefits from medical innovation and groundbreaking research. Further, while no one would question the importance of training healthcare professionals, it is reasonable to consider the nature and scope of that work.[11] Regardless of their tax status, these hospitals receive extensive federal funding through Medicare to administer this training.[12] As explained in the concluding chapter, however, this federal money lacks levers to ensure that national workforce needs—and, more specifically for the current discussion, the needs of the local residents—are met.

Hospitals such as the Cleveland Clinic and Hartford Hospital include research, the flip side of teaching, as one of the major benefits they offer to nearby neighborhoods. Chris Stocking, a dietitian and Cleveland activist, questioned whether it was appropriate for the Clinic to include tens of millions of dollars spent on medical research as a part of their community benefit accounting. When referring to this common practice, Stocking asked: "Does [it] address health in the community? Or are they just looking at medical research in general? Because if they're looking at it in general, I'm not sure the best term for that is a 'community benefit.' It might be a medical benefit, or a benefit to a patient that has a certain disease if a cure is found, but I'm not sure we can really call that *community* benefit." Chris's questions were reasonable ones. The regulations guiding the extent to which hospitals can report research expenditures and educational resources as community benefit disclosures are vague.

Linking training and research *directly* to a hospital's community-based mission, and demonstrating its relevance to communities, can be difficult. A high-level administrator at Anschutz explained that simply being an impressive academic institution was insufficient. Indeed, while he described the work at Anschutz as "educating and training future health professionals and providing tremendous leading-edge research," he also recalled that administrators' initial assumption that residents would "automatically just love" having "this whole academic enterprise" in the area was incorrect. David Crombie, the retired Hartford Hospital physician, understood the community's frustrations. He explained that hospitals have a "commitment to those scholarly endeavors," but acknowledged that communities do not fully grasp the idea of a teaching and research hospital. He believed that communities, rightly, should have an expectation of bringing research to the public. As noted earlier, he understood neighborhood residents as asking the hospital to "do better telling us about our health."

Clearly, internal missions and external expectations, especially community-based expectations, are routinely misaligned. While some aspects of this misalignment could be resolved, or at least contextualized, through better communication, in other cases hospitals and communities simply expect different things from themselves and one another.

PERCEIVED CAPACITY

Hospitals present themselves as accomplished and well-resourced institutions, and this image contributes to the community's perception that hospitals hold the capacity to better support neighborhoods. An employee at the Cleveland Department of Health, for example, lamented that the city's top healthcare institutions hadn't significantly improved community health: "We have four world-class healthcare institutions within our boundaries . . . How can you reconcile the health of the population against some of the really incredible resources that are so close at hand?" Many residents concurred with that sentiment. Elizabeth, a substance abuse prevention worker who lived close to the hospital, described the Cleveland Clinic this way: "They take care of [us], almost from birth to death. We think we know a lot about them, but with all the resources they could put into the community—and I'm not even talking about money, I'm talking about human resources that they could add—the value they could bring into our communities is not happening." Quotes like these, often resting on locals' grasp of hospitals' size and power, show how perceived capacity can drive expectations.

Administrators understood these expectations. According to Gregory, an academic administrator in Cleveland, residents should "hope for and expect a commitment at the highest levels, because this was a community that lacked a lot of resources." In contrast to other participants, however, Gregory felt the Clinic had been able to "satisfy, at some base level, an expectation that [the Clinic] will participate, that they will care, they will make investments in the community." From his perspective, the Clinic has done that, "adequately and quite well."[13]

In the absence of harder data, locals are left to gauge their institution's capacity for community investment through proxies, which can include facilities development and a general sense of long-standing community commitment that we call "fixedness." Earlier chapters include evidence for the first of these proxies: locals observe cranes and backhoes, road closures, and scaffolding around these campuses on a near-daily basis. Less clear, but still in the public's awareness, is the steady regional expansion of hospitals and healthcare systems, especially in suburbs, rural cities, and towns. While locals aren't fully aware of the increasing pressures hospitals and the healthcare industry face broadly, behind-the-scenes rapid growth, mergers, and acquisitions entail substantial risks. Hospitals have, in fact, been absorbed by large healthcare systems, consolidated, and even shuttered.[14]

Locals in our cities generally perceived the development of facilities as a sign of economic vitality. As explained in chapter 3, there was a sense among neighborhood residents that hospital expansion—whether local, regional, or global—was inevitable and boundless. Residents drew comparisons between what they saw and what they felt they were getting in return. When we talked with Warren in a nearby local business he owned that had been almost completely surrounded by new Cleveland Clinic buildings, he remarked, "If they ever stop building . . . If they ever stop expanding, maybe they would, uh, do something here." He added, "I assume they're right at Buckingham Palace, now . . ."

New buildings and facilities can be a source of both great excitement and great disappointment. Hospital marketing campaigns emphasize the benefits of expansion in their community-facing messaging. Those present for the announcements, planning, and building of new medical centers may have a range of expectations. As Mario, an Aurora resident, noted: "At first it seemed like a very shiny, glimmering, full-of-hope sort of situation. 'This looks like a great medical campus. It looks like there's a lot of positivity that's going to come out of this.'" High expectations, however, can give way to disillusionment when Mario and other residents see the resultant development and displacement.[15]

The fixedness of an anchor institution increases community expectations even further, because residents perceive the hospital as both an employment hub and an economic engine. As mentioned in chapter 3, the three hospital campuses are the largest employers in their respective cities. As historian Gabriel Winant argued, however, the rise in prominence of hospitals as major employers and economic engines in U.S. cities is cause for concern as well as celebration. In fact, Winant asserted, the boom in healthcare hiring is a result of both the collapse of industries that once sustained the livelihoods of a comparatively stable working class (Winant's focus is the loss of industry, especially the steel industry, in Western Pennsylvania), and a new economy of ever-growing healthcare institutions that are increasingly dependent on low-wage work disproportionately carried out by women and people of color.[16]

While administrators conveyed hope that their institutions would make a greater investment in their communities, they also expressed a measure of frustration that neighbors, especially more vocal ones, overestimated their hospitals' capacity. At Anschutz, Lilly Marks hoped hospitals "would do more than just provide stellar healthcare, that our presence here would at least help contribute to the lifting of the community." She noted, however, that neighborhood expectations must be calibrated in context: "We can't replace federal programs or state-funded support. It's not who we are; we don't have the resources to do that. I think people have an expectation perhaps greater than the reality in terms of our discretionary income." In another example, Kristen Morris at the Cleveland Clinic said "it's tough" to balance the community's

wide-ranging expectations and the hospital's reality. Drawing from her experiences in community meetings held by the Clinic and radio call-in shows,
Morris concluded, "There are some people who think it is our job to repair
potholes on their streets."

The other side of Morris's pothole reference is a little more nuanced. Listening to local residents, we understood their requests about infrastructure
and roads as being directly related to what they saw as the heavy "wear and
tear" of hospital traffic on neighborhood roads. Indeed, there is merit to the
perception of hospitals as high-traffic hubs.[17] However, expecting hospitals to
compensate for severe urban inequities, infrastructure gaps, and other failures
of the public sector is a heavy burden. The hospital administrators we spoke
with were acutely aware that federal, state, and local fiscal support for their
activities was receding, even as expectations for hospitals to become increasingly involved in an expansive array of health initiatives were on the rise. Thus,
hospitals sometimes act like (and often are) heavyweights, and an unintended
consequence of this posture is the community's expectation that they can offer extensive support to their home cities despite the significant variation in
the skill sets and assets they bring to bear.[18]

Collectively, these are lofty expectations. Hospitals are simply not equipped
to satisfy much of what a given community needs. As a local grants officer in
Cleveland concluded, "A hospital alone can't solve these issues." What, then,
can hospitals do? And what should hospitals do?

Do Formal Obligations Matter?
Values, Hopes, and What Hospitals *Could* and *Should* Do

As mentioned, administrators weren't always eager to talk about the hospital's
formal obligations, preferring to cast their good deeds in a benevolent light.
Hospital leadership and personnel spoke of their institution's charitableness
to the community in broad terms, whether referring to their community as a
neighborhood, a city, a state, a region (as with Children's Hospital Colorado),
or even the world (as with the Cleveland Clinic).[19] This type of "soft" obligation appeared regularly in our conversations with administrators.

Residents rarely mentioned formal obligations either, likely because few
had more than a cursory understanding of IRS requirements and ACA legislation. Those in the nonprofit and healthcare world beyond the hospital were
more inclined to broach the topic directly, primarily because they had both
an understanding of those obligations and an interest in advocating (on be-
half of residents) for hospitals to do more.

The imprecise portrayal of community benefit in the chapter's epigraph is an example of how talk of expectations can shift from specific obligations into the more informal and vague milieu of "values." Administrators preferred such colloquial talk: in their descriptions, hospitals didn't engage in community service to meet legal and regulatory obligations but rather to "benefit the community." In a more candid moment, one hospital administrator said his institution had done some "great things, and it's benefited [our] institutional self-interest. And that's been marginally good or fairly good for the community. But there's still an open question of whether it's a true collaboration for everyone's interest." Such sentiments suggest that community benefit work is often more a byproduct of hospitals' main priorities and less outcomes-oriented work. Thus, while compliance is expected in the face of significant consequences—at least in theory, since oversight is weak—the informal discourse is telling.

Residents spoke at length about hospitals' responsibilities to address broad healthcare needs, specifically access to good care and affordability. For one Auroran, a hospital's responsibility to locals was simply "the responsibility of providing good healthcare." Lori, an Aurora pastor, explained, "If I go to visit someone [at the hospital], I always just say, 'How's it going? Are you getting good care?' and almost always, they say, 'Yes, they've been great to me,' so that's good." Positive clinical experiences can temper expectations framed primarily or entirely by financial considerations. Negative clinical experiences, conversely, prompted some residents to emphasize hospital finances. Other residents specifically mentioned the cost of healthcare services as something they believed hospitals could do something about. Salomé, an Aurora resident who needed a costly medical procedure, said she wished the hospital would see reducing costs for locals as "a way to give back."

Former Aurora mayor Paul Tauer insisted that improving conditions in neighborhoods was not the hospital's responsibility but that of the local government. He concluded, "That's not their job. That's our job." In contrast, Claudia, a nonprofit worker in Cleveland, held a higher standard for hospitals: "I would hope that they wanna give back financially to lower-income neighborhoods, especially since . . . the main campus is located in a low-income neighborhood. So I would hope they would give back to some needs, like financial literacy or housing development. To bring up the areas that surround it." Even without a robust understanding of formal obligations, Lori, the Aurora pastor, articulated expectations that were, in fact, central to hospitals' formal obligations, noting: "I think they could interview the community and ask what the needs are. They could come to our churches; they could go to the nonprofits, especially along Colfax, who are saying, 'We are here to meet [community needs] and here's [what] they are.'" Lori's comment mirrored the required components of CHNAs, and thus her interview is a reminder that CHNAs are not merely legal requirements driving a new turn toward community investments by hospitals and other institutions, but rather are outgrowths of commonsense planning in which hospitals ask local experts for insights into community needs.

Marching in Step

Few residents expected a hospital could or should compensate for decades of urban divestment and neglect. They did, however, believe hospitals should work together in increasingly different, even novel, ways when considering the state of things in the communities just beyond their campus borders.

Take, for example, Sudhir, a Hartfordite who said prevention was an undervalued and implicit goal for hospitals. He saw prevention as a critical way for the hospital to "limit costs and ensure quality of life." He remarked that he wished more neighborhood residents shared that expectation: "I can see other people saying, 'Oh, a hospital doesn't need to be doing that stuff. That's not what it's there for.' But it is, if you want to transition from just being a public institution that provides last-resort emergency care to improving health and well-being overall." Sudhir's thoughts align with emerging beliefs. In discussions about hospitals' growing responsibilities, expectations that hospitals will address prevention are still relatively new.[20] Other residents echoed a broader shift in the discourse of medicine itself, namely that only a focus on population health can ameliorate many of the more entrenched outcomes and disparities plaguing the health of those living in some of the poorest American cities.

Dwight, a nonprofit professional, noted that the ACA's goal was to have "everyone marching in step" with respect to the assessment of community health needs. The question, to extend Dwight's metaphor, is who is conducting this march?

Evidence outlined in earlier chapters showed that residents' and employees' new expectations of hospitals play a large role in promoting economic and racial inclusivity, and in positively impacting goods, services, and previously unavailable community support. Yet the data suggest that few leaders, in either the municipal or corporate worlds, care to take on the mantle of leadership in this area. The result is diffused responsibility in an unclear field of expectations. Passing the buck has become the norm. Instead of an organized effort driven by a clear sense of responsibility, there is an often-diffuse and semi-organized collection of entities each playing a part, while no single organization spearheads the bigger picture. Each entity is hesitant to see themselves as obligated in a larger sense. This is the current scenario despite the many initiatives outlined in previous chapters and despite the growing chorus of voices asking hospitals to not only engage in prevention and community health but to do so in a manner that is both collaborative and inclusive.

One of the reasons for the current situation is that anchor institutions, broadly, are stuck in modes of thinking that don't fully connect with needed community-based work. As Isaac, a professor and physician at University of Colorado Denver, explained, hospitals sometimes confuse population health with "managed care," an approach in which hospitals manage the financial risk of ill health in a way that should improve health outcomes, but which is distinct from direct population health work. He asserted that population health is "about community" and that hospitals and universities should "adopt a different definition for population health" in their missions, although he didn't see that happening just yet.

For Janey, the Cleveland nonprofit health worker with whom we opened chapter 1, a new approach must include any organization that becomes a part of the community taking on a "shared responsibility to the people in whatever capacity or in whichever way that will increase the vitality of that neighborhood or that quality of life there in that neighborhood." Janey understood that this was a difficult position for any single organization, but believed it was the job of city and state government to "create a culture that puts people as the priority first."

Residents who were well versed in community organizing, social change, and urban development, of course, took a stronger, less concessionary position on the matter. Central Connecticut State University professor Reinaldo Rojas held a range of roles in municipal and healthcare organizations in the city and, for example, viewed institutions as playing a larger role in communities: "My expectations would be for far more connectivity, far more of a partnership, of a healing partner, of complete immersion in the neighborhood . . . The neighborhood around [the hospital] should not be one of the poorest neighborhoods in the city; it just makes little sense. It should be one of the richest. It should be a partner in healing, a partner in feeling good, a partner in creating a good part of the city." Rojas added, "If the hospital is a place of healing and a place of well-being, I don't think it's too hard to expect that the well-being of the surrounding community should be part of the mission." For Hartford's Cary Wheaton, the challenge for hospitals and their interest in working "for the good of the community" is that it can be difficult to balance investments in expansion with investments in the neighborhoods surrounding their expanding campuses.

Reinaldo's and Wheaton's expectations in Hartford harmonize with Janey's and others' thoughts about how communities cannot expect such weighty responsibilities to rest solely on the shoulders of hospitals. Yet there remains a tremendous opportunity for hospitals to play a more powerful role, as well as a chance for states to play an important part in compelling them to do so.

Hospitals are understandably wary of setting new and clear expectations. Administrators expressed something akin to what others have observed in the nonprofit sector, a kind of "donor fatigue"—a sense of exhaustion in tackling a specific problem or extending empathy for a particular area.[21] Max, who worked with GUCI, noted that the seeming intractability of poverty in these communities could lead some anchors to "give up" or to point to the lack of progress as evidence that their efforts were unlikely to make a difference. This observation prompted Max to pose a rhetorical question: "How do we continually refresh the work?"

Conclusion: Who Is Responsible for the Health of a Community?

A new paradigm that moves beyond the traditionally cloistered approach of hospitals and toward community-based approaches to population health requires a reworking of mission and shared expectations. In fact, both the formal and informal concern with "community benefit" assumes that the original mission of hospitals—meeting the basic healthcare needs of a population—has already been challenged. Though it is unlikely that these largely change-averse institutions will move toward this new paradigm with any urgency, the emerging expectations we observed among residents and even administrators suggest that the forces at work are unlikely to be reversed in the coming years. As residents made clear, the shifting of people's perceptions of hospitals beyond earlier paradigms suggests these institutions are newly available as assets, with renewed creative potential, to those interested in promoting population health.

The specific question being negotiated, after decades of efforts to increase access to direct medical services for individuals, concerns who is responsible for the health of a community. The preceding chapters make clear that neighborhood residents often believe specific issues should be addressed, and expect their local hospitals to help address them. At the same time, locals tend to be pragmatic about community benefit and accept that hospitals' internal missions may not align with neighborhood expectations. This outlook persists, moreover, regardless of the size or perceived economic standing of a medical institution. Even as some hospital neighbors are vocal advocates for hospitals' engagement in community benefit, there is a palpable acceptance, resignation even, that limited hospital engagement in communities, beyond providing clinical care, is simply the state of things in American medicine. The next chapter offers concrete ideas to begin to move us beyond this great impasse in American urban health.

6

Six Policy Ideas for Communities and Hospitals

I think we have pretty good legislation, but it's up to the IRS to enforce it—and to deny [hospitals] tax-exempt status if they're not doing their job . . . If you do that once you're going to send a message to the whole profession. That'll straighten things out.
SENATOR CHUCK GRASSLEY[1]

A largely unnoticed but consequential thing happened in the 2019 Democratic presidential primary: Pete Buttigieg, former mayor of South Bend, Indiana, identified hospital billing practices as an important part of why the American healthcare system was unsustainable.[2] This moment was noteworthy in part because it was a clear departure from the more familiar criticisms limited to insurance companies and the pharmaceutical industry, but also because in making hospital pricing part of his larger healthcare vision, Buttigieg—who would go on to serve as President Biden's Secretary of Transportation—risked angering powerful stakeholders, especially the American Hospital Association and its army of lobbyists. Politicians have long attempted to avoid direct conflict with the hospital industry.

Given the respect many Americans have for hospitals, including hospitals in the larger critique of U.S. healthcare and urban planning can be risky political business. Yet it is becoming increasingly clear that a sober analysis of the complex and central role hospitals play within American cities must be part of conversations about improving health outcomes.

We opened this book with a troubling paradox: How can American cities house some of the most innovative and well-capitalized healthcare institutions in the world, yet be home to health outcomes worse than those in many non-industrialized nations? This mystery reflects an even more troubling fact about the U.S. healthcare system, namely that, despite spending more per capita on healthcare than most major, industrialized nations, Americans have very little to show for it in terms of life expectancy and quality of life. The fundamental reason these poor outcomes persist in the face of significant healthcare resources is that U.S. communities remain profoundly unequal, with extensive residential segregation and limited opportunities for social mobility. While social inequality is almost certainly the foundation of America's poor bill of health, direct actions to reshape social life remain unpalatable to many Americans. Instead, the U.S. prefers a somewhat unique approach to improving community health. While in most industrialized countries, the government both organizes health services and provides direct investments to improve social life, the U.S. has favored a partnership approach in which private businesses, especially hospitals, fill the role of providing healthcare and making neighborhood investments to improve community health.

Given this scenario, we end this book by offering six concrete policy ideas—some quite specific, others more general, some primarily municipal, others at the state and federal levels—that could incentivize and even force hospitals to undertake work that would improve community health outcomes. We argue that in the absence of larger political changes that directly address health inequality, these policies constitute pragmatic, local, and place-based ways to improve health outcomes and, most importantly, close persistent gaps between racial/ethnic groups and across socioeconomic lines. As explained in the previous chapters, for myriad reasons, hospitals are positioned to play an important, even transformative role in promoting access to care and addressing health disparities in urban neighborhoods. While health improvement faces considerable hurdles in the U.S., an outsized share of healthcare dollars is located within hospitals as well as the larger campuses and health systems of which they are a part. For this reason, and in recognition of the parts that they've played in urban inequalities, we still believe hospitals—perhaps more than almost any other U.S. institution—have the potential to address the underlying conditions that allow poor health outcomes and health disparities to persist.

Building on the landscape of assets, opportunities, and challenges detailed in preceding chapters, we now explain how hospitals can play a larger and more sustained role in health promotion, disease prevention, and addressing social determinants of health. The focus of this final chapter is the identification of mechanisms—ranging from the establishment of financial resources and incentives, to culture change within institutions, to more explicit policies—to drive health improvement.

Changing Culture: From Funding to Organizational Norms

While policy has the potential to be a key driver moving hospitals to more meaningful action to improve health outcomes in communities, the ground is shifting in ways that incentivize hospitals to do more—or adjust their focus—to align with currents in population health. Two key developments have incentivized activity in these policy areas: 1) the increasing availability of funds for undertaking transformative community-based work, and 2) broader institutional and cultural norms that shape, and in some instances embed, the kind of expectations hospitals have of themselves.

FUNDING STREAMS

Money talks, of course, so funding will be essential to hospitals' ability to engage community benefit and building work more fully, or to deepen existing commitments and projects. As we have already suggested, we should expect hospitals to simply spend more of their existing revenue to support this work, and efforts should be intensified to push them to do this. "Fair-share deficits" should be cause for civic and moral outrage. There is also, as expected, a growing and substantial base of nonprofit and specifically foundation funding for this kind of work, and those resources should be fully leveraged. As outlined in chapter 4, foundations played central roles in shaping the dynamics in all three cities,[3] and when we interviewed people in each of these organizations, they saw themselves primarily as conveners, bringing anchor institutions together with locals to work on community development. Such funding creates opportunities for meaningful collaboration between anchor institutions and a range of local organizations, including the types of organizations discussed in previous chapters. Anchor institutions should wield their resources and significant expertise with grants to assist local community groups in applying for, administering, and assessing grant-funded community development work.[4]

On a larger scale, the federal government can use its granting ability to encourage anchor institutions to address health disparities in meaningful ways while democratizing decision-making processes within communities. Specifically, place-based grants could encourage a range of activities consistent with anchor institutions' aims, but instead of targeting services and programs, such grants must target specific locations, making them a promising tool for addressing the kind of challenges examined in earlier chapters.[5]

With hospitals, such grants should include requirements that anchor institutions establish meaningful partnerships with local organizations and include extensive community input in planning.[6] Despite formal requirements to solicit neighborhood residents' input to identify local health needs, community benefit programming has at times undermined a place-based approach by allowing anchors to invest in priorities other than those identified by the community or to invest in different communities altogether. Similarly, formal rules governing community benefit have required little or no formal consultation with communities regarding the implementation of community building initiatives. As a corrective to this shortcoming, new and innovative grants could earmark funds for projects conducted in a genuinely community-engaged manner.

The sheer number of areas in which hospital decisions impact communities highlights the need for meaningful collaborative bodies, such as community advisory boards. An even more impactful approach is to take a page from federal legislation governing community health centers, which requires formal neighborhood representation on boards. Specifically, certification by the Health Resources and Services Administration requires that a "majority [at least 51 percent] of the health center board members must be patients served by the health center."[7] Whatever the specific manifestation of this policy approach, the core focus is the democratization of hospital decision-making in areas that impact surrounding communities. External funding should be attached to requirements for the increased democratization of decision-making in areas that impact, directly or indirectly, communities.

These funding mechanisms would serve as a welcome supplement to broader changes in the financing of healthcare itself, in which many hospitals are now engaged. The move toward so-called value-based healthcare purchasing, for example, gradually incentivizes higher-quality care and quality improvement by attaching lower reimbursement rates and penalties to preventable emergency room readmissions, thus encouraging hospitals to connect patients with a medical home to ensure good access to primary and specialty care.[8] But beyond their potential to change the financing of healthcare services and improve value,[9] "risk-bearing" models could be leveraged to nudge hospitals toward more of a preventive model, especially regarding investments in addressing upstream factors that could lessen the need for expensive direct medical services that have long been the bread and butter of the traditional hospital. The key to these arrangements is that hospitals and hospital systems must take responsibility for outcomes, assuming risks to position themselves for rewards. The effect of this approach is a renewed incentive to invest in prevention.[10]

Additional federal, state, and private nonprofit funding streams can provide hospitals with potentially powerful tools for achieving goals attached to seemingly intractable problems (e.g., revitalizing housing stock without inducing gentrification and offering abatements to promote environmental health). That the incentives and penalties included in the larger industry dynamics of such a shift would likely spur creative, community-oriented work similar to the projects discussed in this book is an added benefit.

NEW NORMS WITHIN AND BEYOND HOSPITALS

Establishing new norms will make community benefit and building, as both formal and informal expectations, a mainstay of community-based health and urban development. As shown in the prior chapters, many, though certainly not all, hospitals are undergoing just such a change in dynamic interplay with their surrounding communities.

As we've noted, education in medicine and other health professions reflects these normative shifts, which is a promising sign that a generational effect may be underway.[11] Educators and practitioners have a growing sense that medical practice requires a curricular change to include skills in healthcare finance, epidemiology, population health, health policy, and other areas. More broadly, and compounded by experiences from the COVID-19 pandemic, there is a growing consensus in the scholarly literature that improving health outcomes and reducing disparities will require much more engagement with the social determinants of health than currently occurs.[12] All of these developments put pressure on healthcare institutions, including hospitals, to rework their guiding philosophies of both direct patient care and community engagement.

Though bottom-up culture change is important, culture change in healthcare must also entail strong and unequivocal leadership. While we have described mostly superficial mission statements and fleeting events bringing about some change in communities, as Gregory from Cleveland explained, it is clearly also the case that leadership is important: "The leadership group at the top sets the tone, sends the message, and sets the execution. And I say 'leadership group' because there are lots of individual leaders that understand what needs to be done, but until they put in place people around them that also understand and can execute, it becomes just the leader themselves. They may or may not get traction." Meaningful leadership is important because community benefit and community building work has potentially sweeping financial implications, which creates a need for CEOs, CFOs, board members, and others to clarify that an institution not only values this work in principle but regards it as part of its financial model.

Earlier chapters highlighted the proliferation of community-facing positions in hospital administration, from vice presidents for community health and engagement to neighborhood relations managers and similar positions, and we talked with many people in these positions for this book. Clearly, however, commitments to population health within institutions are uneven, with champions and skeptics often residing in the same departments. This diversity of perspectives and priorities within institutions makes leadership essential and underscores the importance of implementing clear internal policies and procedures that remind employees at various levels that community-facing work is a key part of the hospital's mission.

Because of this diversity of views, it is difficult to talk about "the hospital" or "the institution" in broad terms. As Richard explained, "Even the best innovative examples are often disconnected from overarching narratives." He underscored how institutions work at cross-purposes, and institutionalization is the only path to maintain any "initial burst of excitement, energy, [and] possibility." As we have shown throughout this book, community members are often frustrated that the establishment of these norms appears to be taking hold at a glacial pace. Many times, at least some of a hospital's employees are unaware that such organizational shifts and on-the-ground work is occurring at all, which suggests that, if institutions are serious about making this kind of work part of their institutional culture, transparency and clarity in internal communications is a place to start.

Policies to Move Hospitals toward Community-Based Health

To ensure that such "initial bursts" of energy and excitement gain a foothold, therefore, external stimuli are necessary. While internal culture change is important, and can be transformative, experience suggests external pressure also compels hospitals into action. While the focus in this book has been on the three cities we examined closely, every community, despite sharing in some commonalities, will have a unique origin story for this kind of work, with their individual histories, challenges, and injustices—but also unique assets and respectable champions of this work—shaping the specific articulation of the collective life they will live with and alongside their respective communities.

One of the curious dynamics of the current state of community benefit is that, absent meaningful external forces, institutions that want to do this work will, and those that don't want to do this work will do as little as possible. Few institutions do nothing, of course, and even those that do the minimum pay lip service to population health. It is therefore necessary to consider how policy, as either a main driver of or supplement to ongoing work, can improve outcomes and address disparities. Based on the research presented here, we identify six critical points for policy intervention: EMTALA; health professions (including medical) education; community benefit provisions; transparency and accounting; considerations of space; and campus policing.

The optimistic view of well-meaning hospitals whose leadership and rank and file are staked in being positive forces within communities must be balanced by a sober analysis of institutions and organizations that change only

when incentives are correctly aligned or they are compelled to do so. Each of
the preceding chapters pointed to policies that could restructure how hospitals engage their surrounding communities. To offer a clearer picture of how
existing policy frameworks could be better leveraged in pursuit of hospital
efforts to improve population health while reducing disparities, we suggest
that the following policy ideas are potentially essential answers to the questions that animated this book. While it is not an exhaustive set of policy recommendations, we believe this is a unique collection of ideas, largely unseen
in the literature. In presenting these policy ideas, however, we do not intend
to advance a one-size-fits-all approach, but rather a suite of adjustments that
we believe are attainable because they attempt to capitalize on existing policy
frameworks. Indeed, most of these ideas would not require passage of major
legislation but could be carried out through executive orders and administrative rules on the federal as well as state level.

REVISITING EMTALA

As discussed in chapter 4, emergency departments are important contact
zones between hospitals and communities. Since it became federal law in
1986, the Emergency Medical Treatment and Labor Act (EMTALA) has as-
sured the provision of direct medical care by EDs and the stabilization and
non-abandonment of patients, as in the case of Eduardo Franco Ramirez, the
Auroran who received care, though only minimally, at University of Colorado Hospital. Amending EMTALA to move hospitals toward prevention will
be crucial if we wish them to be more meaningful participants in community health, especially to address disparities. Just as importantly, however, the
federal government should leverage EMTALA to ensure that immigrants—
including undocumented immigrants—can receive meaningful care in nonprofit, public, and even for-profit medical facilities where federal resources
are present.

EMTALA expresses "deeply held social values and beliefs," and is a rare
example of a law that responds, though in a limited way, to widespread complaints that American healthcare fails to consider the needs of patients.[13] The
act, however, is a relic of earlier thinking about hospitals, wherein the concern
was primarily with acute needs, with no emphasis on prevention. Expanding the legislation to include preventive care would help to reposition and
de-densify hospital EDs and their waiting rooms, as upstream engagements
should reduce emergent care visits. Further, an important consideration
within the framework of the questions posed in this book, from a spatial perspective, is that EMTALA requirements concern only those patients who come

through hospital doors, whether under their own power or by ambulance. Nothing in EMTALA concerns the community or the upstream effects that lead to ED visits. This legislation, therefore, is a necessary but shortsighted approach to health.

Perhaps most glaringly, as its name suggests, EMTALA is expressly focused on emergencies instead of prevention and does not require that hospitals, whether nonprofit or public, reach outward into communities to prevent the very ED admissions the law requires that they make. The result is that the key point of contact between the city and hospital is barely a part of conversations about population health and population health management, except as an example of the shortcomings of the U.S. healthcare system.[14] As noted earlier, however, an underlying aim of the "value-based" healthcare contracting that some policy experts hope will replace "fee-for-service" models is to reduce emergency department visits. As hospitals increasingly become responsible for health outcomes in defined areas beyond hospital walls, they are likely to think of their emergency departments not as the sole contact zone, but rather as part of a continuum of interaction with communities. Yet as these changes in the financing of healthcare potentially generate significant change in population health, such outcomes remain secondary concerns.

It's important to note that financial incentives are necessary but insufficient. While community stakeholders cannot leverage hospitals' federal funding without limit, it is worth considering policy mechanisms that could be attached to EMTALA to engender improvements in community and population health. For example, instead of depending on a turn to value-based healthcare creating incentives for hospitals to look upstream and invest in prevention, EMTALA could simply be amended to require them to do so. As part of the CHNA process, for example, data collection regarding the most common reasons for ED admission could be linked to an implementation plan for addressing the causes of those admissions. Care would have to be taken, of course, to ensure that such requirements didn't simply create a moral hazard in which hospitals misreported such admissions. Oversight and periodical audits would be essential. But whatever the ultimate shape of such a requirement, the policy aim would be to update EMTALA to prevent ED admissions substantively instead of merely addressing—in a notoriously inefficient way—the downstream effects of poor community health investments.

REORIENTING GRADUATE MEDICAL EDUCATION

A second policy recommendation is to mandate community-based health education in medical training. The previous chapter noted that many hospitals wish for a greater appreciation of their efforts as teaching hospitals. Though many hospitals fund medical residents as part of their operating budgets, Medicare is the largest single payer for the training of medical residents in the U.S., totaling $9.5 billion annually.[15] As with Medicaid and Medicare reimbursement rates, there is considerable debate, and many unanswered questions, about whether hospitals benefit financially, lose money, or break even on the medical residents they fund with federal money. Certainly, the question is more complicated than any of these individual answers. As with hospital pricing and other aspects of the U.S. healthcare system, transparency is a perennial debate, and there is good reason to wonder if graduate medical education (GME) funding is adequately serving the public in ways that justify the billions spent on training.[16]

Teaching hospitals receive billions each year to not only support the education of the emerging healthcare workforce, but also provide care to patients in their hospitals. Increasingly, this training also serves as a feeder for the hospital systems housing GME programs, suggesting these training programs can be understood as federally subsidized workforce development. While many hospitals argue that they currently subsidize the training of residents, Medicare also subsidizes patient care, generating untold amounts of revenue. All the while, critics note transparency is lacking in the current GME system, with many hospitals making it all but impossible to know how much they receive in "indirect payments" as part of the GME payment schema.

All these factors raise the question, similar to the one we posed regarding EMTALA, of whether the federal government could attach Medicare funding to incentives that would nudge hospitals to become more community-minded in their educational work. Training clinicians to perform key clinical tasks is of course a foundation of their education, but if U.S. healthcare is to evolve into a preventive and population health-focused model that addresses health disparities and chronic illness, the training of healthcare professionals themselves must be part of the overall strategy. Leveraging the extensive federal investments in GME must be a part of this effort.

Throughout this book, we have suggested that hospital organizations would do well to learn more about their communities, particularly because this knowledge is a precondition to understanding those communities' health needs and fostering local partnerships. This community orientation should become part of their legacy as teaching hospitals. Rare cases in which medical residency programs have included neighborhood histories in training for new physicians provide possible guidance.[17] However, few U.S. hospitals include a historical perspective on the hospital's own place within the community as part of their orientation of new employees.[18] New employees enter their positions without a historical understanding of their communities. Most training, un-fortunately, comprises limited "field trips" or one-off experiences.[19] But more than learning about specific communities, healthcare professions training should include a focus on fostering what is often called "structural compe-tence" to eliminate persistent race- and class-based health disparities in the U.S. As Jonathan Metzl notes, there are serious gaps in current training, each of which concerns the social and structural factors underlying health.[20]

A steady growth in community-based training programs gives reason for optimism, but such programs remain primarily within the relatively cloistered environs of community health centers.[21] The absence of residency programs that help future physicians and other health professionals to not only encounter neighborhood residents from a clinical perspective, but also understand the upstream effects leading to their health conditions, makes it difficult to fathom health disparities; further, this absence seems to undercut attempts to carry out community benefit initiatives and forge partnerships with residents. Perhaps the most glaring deficiency is that few hospitals engage with local histories as part of their investments in their cities, connecting history to epidemiology. This oversight hamstrings community-facing initiatives billed as increasing ac-cess to healthcare on both the individual patient and population levels.

Leveraging Medicare cannot, of course, be the only strategy for addressing the relationship at the heart of this study. As historians of policy know, Medi-care shaped emergency department policy, graduate medical education, and other aspects of the healthcare system, but as a matter of convenience, not as careful and intentional policy design.[22] As conversations continue in the U.S. about the prospects of larger, more sweeping healthcare reform—including the pursuit of "Medicare for All," or a similar national healthcare plan—the re-sulting plan will provide further leverage regarding both the community/ED relationship and medical education.

BOLSTERING COMMUNITY BENEFIT PROVISIONS

As explained in the introduction, the ACA's community benefit provisions were an animating reason for writing this book. Yet, considering the vague regulatory framework, it appears Congress never intended the ACA's com-munity benefit provisions to be transformative, at least not on a large scale. We view this as a missed opportunity in need of further clarification.

There are signs that hospitals take community benefit seriously, of course. Notably, for example, in 2018 the American Hospital Association released a re-source guide entitled "Protecting Your Hospital's Non-Profit Status: Compli-ance with the Affordable Care Act and Final IRS Section 501(r) Regulations," which described the procedures for compliance and consequences for non-compliance, but did not address broader contexts, such as generous public subsidies and neighborhood residents' expectations that often sit in tension with hospitals' finances.[23]

As this chapter's epigraph indicates, concerns about oversight and enforcement appear warranted. As the chairman of the U.S. Senate Committee on Finance during periods of Republican majority, Iowa Senator Chuck Grassley has stressed the importance of ensuring that "tax-exempt hospitals are fulfilling the standards for serving communities and low-income patients as required by law."[24] But the pervasive sense that oversight is lacking aligns with a 2020 Government Accountability Office finding that the "IRS was unable to provide evidence that it conducts reviews related to hospitals' community benefits because it does not have codes to track such audits."[25]

Formal compliance with federal law is a minimum requirement that most institutions take seriously. As the American Hospital Association explains the consequences: "Failure to meet [ACA] requirements can have significant consequences, ranging from the $50,000 excise tax for each hospital facility that fails to perform a timely community health needs assessment and adopt a corresponding implementation plan, to taxing all of a hospital facility's revenue for one or more years, to loss of exempt status for that hospital organization and for the interest on its bonds."[26]

And yet, the variance in institutional approaches to community benefit raises questions about the effectiveness of these legally sanctioned penalties. For every example of engaged institutions devoting significant time and resources to communities via sustained efforts to improve population health, many more do substantially less. The primary driver of hospital engagement in these practices seems to be less community benefit regulations than hospitals' missions to improve health and other local expectations to engage in community improvement.

Community benefit compliance lacks both compelling enough carrots and sufficiently fearsome sticks.[27] At least one hospital has lost its nonprofit status for lack of compliance with community benefit requirements, and there have been a few attempts on the part of municipal leaders to chasten hospitals: the mayor of Pittsburgh unsuccessfully suing a hospital to challenge its status in 2013; a New Jersey judge ordering a tax-exempt hospital to pay property taxes.[28] There appears to be little will on the part of the federal government to enforce any requirements for specific types of engagement or dollars spent.[29]

Notably, even early in the Trump administration, when full ACA repeal by the Republican Congress appeared all but inevitable, few-to-no Americans seemed to understand that even lesser-known provisions within the ACA's expansive text—such as the community benefit provisions—would be undone by ACA repeal. Those provisions will probably remain poorly understood among the public. There is a real question about what the prime movers are in the evolution of hospital/community relations. While few Americans know the ACA contains rules regarding community benefit, it is plausible that trends toward engagement wouldn't have changed much had the ACA been repealed. As shown earlier, hospitals doing this work are largely responding to, rather than driving, shifts in expectations and broader changes in medicine and healthcare. In this light, it seems more accurate to view the ACA's community benefit provisions as an effect instead of a cause. Lackluster oversight of ACA's community benefit provisions reinforces this assessment. Further, hospitals are not required to invest in the needs identified in their community health needs assessments, but rather are given flexibility to align new programs with institutional resources and expertise.[30]

Our research points to an urgent need for policymakers, advocates, scholars, and others to pressure the IRS to sharpen its expectations of nonprofit hospitals with regard to the penalties authorized by the ACA. In particular, there is a need for more specific guidance on the types of activities that count as community benefit.[31] Congress appears to have underspecified some community benefit rules to retain wide definitional latitude, possibly in hopes of not arousing the ire of hospitals over these provisions.[32] In effect, however, the underspecification left hospitals without adequate guidance, not only on the matter of defining "community," but also regarding the preparation of implementation plans in partnership with their communities to ensure that priority health needs are identified and addressed adequately. Hospital groups are likely to push back against expanded requirements, preferring that community health investments remain voluntary, but in some cases additional direction might be perceived as providing clarity to help institutions remain compliant.

In addition, as part of its approach toward ensuring that nonprofit hospitals serve communities, Congress should implement additional oversight to curb hospitals' aggressive debt collection tactics (known in legal parlance as "extraordinary collection actions"). Such tactics, which have continued even through the COVID-19 pandemic, hurt communities, especially communities of color.[33] Though the ACA community benefit requirements included restrictions on debt collection, increased oversight is needed. Specifically, the ACA requires hospitals to forgo liens on homes, lawsuits, or arrests, among other tactics, and to determine whether patients are eligible for financial aid before undertaking debt collection. It is reasonable to ask whether there is any effective oversight of these federal community benefit requirements, aside from rare and marginal cases.[34]

48CHAPTER SIX

Weak or absent community benefit oversight is one result of federal policies that tried to nudge hospitals through tax reporting obligations without arousing concern from their well-funded lobbies. The National Academy for State Health Policy made recommendations about a role for states as well.[35] For example, Illinois and Utah have tied expectations for community benefit spending to the equivalent of property taxes not paid to the state because of nonprofit status, while Pennsylvania's Institutions of Purely Public Charity Act outlines the conditions under which nonprofits, including hospitals, can claim tax-exempt status.[36] Other states have mandated partnerships with public health departments or required hospitals to align their community benefit programs with state health improvement plans in an attempt to integrate hospitals into larger public health networks.

The National Academy for State Health Policy noted that states can make conditions for community benefit part of their licensing process. The organization highlighted, for example, the case of one of the states featured in this book, Connecticut, which like the majority of states uses "certificate of need" (CON) laws to limit the development of new healthcare facilities and reduce duplication, including to ensure that community investments are demonstrably meaningful when healthcare organizations are undergoing major changes. Connecticut's CON process is designed to ask more from hospitals engaged in mergers and acquisitions, ensuring that new owners and their companies are invested in charitable work for their communities.

Whatever form these policies take, states must take greater responsibility, especially considering the lack of federal oversight. States are in many ways better positioned to observe and understand the actual charitable and community benefit dispositions of hospitals and their impact on local and state health outcomes. Of course, hospitals and hospital systems often have tremendous leverage over state legislators and executives, as they do over federal policymakers, which may challenge these and other changes to the community benefit process.

TRANSPARENCY AND ACCOUNTING

While revisiting EMTALA, addressing medical education, and expanding community benefit requirements are concerned with rethinking and revising policies and practices, it is important to stay focused on the more general need for hospitals to provide greater transparency for communities and those who advocate for communities. As noted earlier in the book, hospitals are notoriously tight-lipped about their inner workings. Despite the public availability of tax documents for nonprofits, this tendency toward secrecy is a significant roadblock for social accountability. If hospitals wish to benefit from nonprofit status, they must see themselves as public entities with public responsibilities, which includes allowing communities to easily learn how they operate, what they charge, and what their actual policies are—from healthcare access to policies regarding hiring, procurement, and engagements with municipal and other entities.

Comments recounted throughout this book suggest an important question: Would it be preferable for nonprofit hospitals to simply become for-profit entities in order to avoid the transparency that is required as formal partners with federal and, increasingly, state governments? In a 2017 interview, the journalist Dan Diamond asked former Cleveland Clinic CEO Toby Cosgrove about nonprofit status. The moment is worth considering in full:

COSGROVE: I think that we have more than fulfilled our duties as a tax-exempt organization, not to mention education. Have you visited the high school here, recently, that we are participants in—John Hay High School? Which now has 100 percent of their kids going to college?

DIAMOND: And that's because of a Clinic initiative?

COSGROVE: Yeah, it is. We're part of it.

DIAMOND: I have talked to folks in the city who say that there could be more though. If the Clinic was taxed, that is tens of millions of dollars more into local school districts, and I think from the year you started as head of the Clinic there has been a focus—Washington, Chuck Grassley asked the Clinic to testify on its role in the community. Local regulators have eyed the clinic for tax-exempt dollars. It doesn't feel like this is ever going to totally go away. Would the Clinic ever be interested in a payment in lieu of taxes program like has been done in Boston or other cities?

COSGROVE: As soon as they start doing the same thing with the churches, and the Salvation Army, and the Red Cross, and all the other tax-exempt organizations, we'd be happy to do our part.[37]

Notably, Cosgrove makes a direct comparison between the hospital system he led and organizations such as churches and the Salvation Army and the Red Cross. Indeed, the latter two organizations have deep pockets, but does the analogy hold? As shown throughout this book, hospitals, with their large footprint, healthcare mission, and penchant for expansion, are different entities altogether. One key difference is that churches, the Salvation Army, the Red Cross, and other tax-exempt organizations are not at the scale of the multibillion-dollar healthcare industry, most of which is for-profit in the U.S.

The proposition of nonprofit hospitals who fail to invest adequately in community health becoming for-profit businesses has some upsides. Such entities could deduct community benefit and other charitable work from their taxable inflows; this approach would presumably offer a cleaner mode of accounting. Or, perhaps, the Anschutz Medical Center provides a model, showing that hospitals can also consider pursuing status as a public entity, which would largely end the conversation about "fair-share deficits," shifting the conversation to other areas, such as institutional commitments to equity, community health, and charity.

As shown earlier, these tensions regarding community benefit do not only exist between hospitals and communities, but within healthcare institutions themselves. Hospital administrators made it clear that their organizations were having these conversations internally, with important divisions regarding the future of the hospital organization. Whether hospitals can simultaneously balance community health engagement with increasing sophistication in medical technology and treatment remains unclear. These responses from administrators illustrate the complexity of both understanding urban health disparities and determining how hospital organizations can improve poor health outcomes. But even within these conversations, there is a tension between the forward face—the shiny facade of branding and public relations—and the messier, more complicated realities within hospital walls and board rooms.

Perhaps more than any other policy area we have described, transparency and publicly accessible accounting are likely to require external levers on both the state and federal levels. Given such changes in the financing of healthcare, especially alternative payment models, there simply is no internal incentive for hospitals to open their books in a way that allows communities to understand exactly what policies and procedures exist, as well as the decisions that dictate the way hospitals interact with communities, especially in the key contact zones we have explored.

RE-ENVISIONING SPACE

Although some administrators felt otherwise, many of the interviewees viewed urban hospitals as imposing fortifications. Health policy should also re-envision hospitals' spaces, requiring hospitals to be more accessible to their communities. Re-envisioning space requires taking a macro-level view of hospitals as 24-hour-a-day, 7-day-a-week urban institutions. Chris, a local planner in Cleveland, said that "big, single-use" facilities that only operate during the day "don't really create a holistic, healthy neighborhood." Thus, "Meds" could aspire to be less like corporate commuter workplaces, and instead draw inspiration from "Eds." Some urban universities and colleges in the U.S. are, in fact, devising new ways to turn their traditionally single-use campuses into more lively multi-use spaces without contributing to the pervasive commercialization of urban spaces.[38] City, county, and state negotiations can leverage public investments and other arrangements to require more multi-use planning.

Such an approach would have to include emergency department waiting rooms as well, which will always be the 24-hour point of contact for hospitals. EDs must keep this important role, not just for emergency healthcare but also for access to air conditioning and heat, social services, and safety.[39] A more important task is to understand EDs as sociologically complex spaces containing clues about communities, health disparities and needs, and other non-clinical phenomena.[40] Conversely, scholars and health planners alike should critically evaluate—and contextualize within the broader consideration of hospitals' community-mindedness—elite VIP suites, high-end cafeterias, and swanky conference rooms, to determine the accessibility of these spaces.

More broadly, administrators, hospital planners, and landscape architects can consider the design of medical campuses. In the preceding chapters, we flagged how hospitals have invested resources in not only the cutting-edge architectural design of facilities, but also landscapes and external spaces, including community-based health centers and clinics, located beyond hospital campus borders and "in" communities. These developments are just as important as, or at least a powerful supplement to, rethinking the use of spaces within hospitals and medical centers. Because local municipalities have their own requirements regarding traffic, parking, structure height, greenspace, and other aspects of contemporary urban design, zoning boards, municipal leaders, and other stakeholders should pressure healthcare institutions at these vital junctures, whenever they can. While it is possible that new policy will be necessary, community conversations driven by nonprofits and neighborhood groups, and even in some instances activism, should press municipalities and communities to expect more from their hospitals, and to approach the expansion and other practices of hospitals and medical centers as a community concern.

Given that many healthcare institutions receive generous accommodations from cities when they expand, there is a largely untapped source of municipal power that could force hospitals and medical institutions to take community needs seriously as part of their long-term institutional planning. There is a persistent sense in the urban planning literature, for example, that municipalities often award tax abatements too easily, without considering the broader expansionary contexts in which entities operate.[41] In 2016, the

Governmental Accounting Standards Board (the nonprofit that sets accounting and financial reporting standards for state and local governments) established new standards addressing transparency in tax abatements.[42] But,
as a local Ohio policy watchdog noted, it "will take a strong commitment by
public officials and residents alike to make the most of the opportunity."[43]
And while a stronger commitment on the part of elected officials is key to de-
manding more from anchor institutions as they grow and expand, this commitment should be reinforced by demands from communities.

Given the complexity of these institutions and their various community
and municipal arrangements, it will be important to use multiple levers, such
as making inclusive and community-minded spatial planning part of nonprofit hospitals' and medical centers' legal obligations when renovations and
expansions are undertaken. Policymakers could devise levers irrespective of
the presence of tax abatements and other municipal arrangements, though it
is also true that policymakers could leverage these arrangements to a greater
extent than they have to date. Such requirements would serve as useful supple-
ments—and potentially powerful ones, at that—to the emerging cultural shifts
within healthcare described herein. Richard, a nonprofit advocate for the democratization of communities' economies, noted that the focus must be on
"developing new models and pathways from . . . theory to action that can both
engage institutions, and also catalyze the ecosystem needed to build community wealth and drive that systemic change."

One such movement to re-envision space is through advocating for the
well-known strategy of creating community land trusts.[44] As the data in chapter 3 show, there is significant concern among residents about property development, and some nonprofits are eager to work with anchor institutions to
address neighborhood affordable housing crises and provide mixed-income
housing in their communities. Bon Secours Mercy Health, a Catholic healthcare system with footprints in seven states, is funding just such a program,
and policymakers should look to that example, and others, for ways to use
space and build community wealth.[45]

The larger point is that meaningful community input should be taken seriously when decisions are made about a wide range of spatial considerations.
These decisions include, among others, the physical connectivity between the
campus and its communities; the use of community spaces within hospital walls;
how the hospital communicates with these communities in an ongoing and
substantive manner, including around both access to healthcare services and
the evolution of the campus; the establishment of signage and interpretive
and translational services; and planning for catastrophic events, from natural
disasters to pandemics to mass shootings. In general, hospitals, as community

resources, should have plans in place for utilizing their facilities and mobilizing their workforces in different eventualities.

Considering the policing practices discussed in chapter 4, a sixth policy direction is the establishment of a process for tracking and overseeing the work of private security forces on hospital campuses. One relatively easy and potentially effective policy development would be, as suggested in chapter 4, to create a kind of "Clery Act for Hospitals" that would track crime and related issues on hospital campuses, including those not affiliated with universities (the current Clery Act is framed around universities). New regulations should go beyond current reporting requirements, which emphasize hospitals' responsibilities to report crimes they suspect within the course of providing medical treatment to patients. Similarly, better reporting to illuminate how private security forces interact with communities could be made a condition of federal funding and tax-exemption. While some reporting exists,[46] stronger requirements should take a genuinely community-oriented approach, with reports detailing crimes committed on medical campuses themselves—both inside and beyond hospital walls—and containing information that contextualizes those crimes within hospital/community relations. In the case of hospitals and medical centers, federal nonprofit laws could be leveraged, though protections must be implemented to prevent such data from being used to harm vulnerable communities (e.g., identifying undocumented persons as either victims or perpetrators). Chapter 4 also flagged how Cleveland's University Circle private security forces were not receiving needed oversight via civilian review boards, despite agreements made with the city.

As hospitals develop policies around greater integration into communities, they should apply the same general philosophy broadly to the many elements of their work. Regarding medical campus security staff, policies governing their day-to-day work should reflect the values of this new approach to healthcare institutions, drawing on the latest and best practices of community policing.

Conclusion: Population Health and the Twenty-First-Century Hospital

On an outdoor walk, Brian Hyde, a conservationist in Aurora, talked with us about a more environmental approach to health, mentioning that the history of medical care in Denver was modeled on the image of tuberculosis sanatoriums in the Alps. He said that he harbored an "idealized image" of a hospital:

> If I were building a university—and in a sense, you're building a mini-university with a medical school—I would want the same things. If there's streams and topography and green spaces, I'd want them integrated and connected and let anybody on their lunch break enjoy that by stepping out the door and there it is. And whether you're a patient or an employee or a visitor, that is simply one more "public facility" that engages you to meet the natural setting in which your city is located or in which the particular campus that you're on, the medical campus, is located.

He commented that hospitals in Denver aren't woven into the geographical landscape in this way.

At the start of this book, we posited that hospitals can and should play a more central role in rethinking and promoting population health. As we noted, however, the early history of U.S. hospitals was characterized by a sense that they were mostly dreary places to avoid—and specifically places where the poor went to die—while in more recent times they are perceived as intimidating urban behemoths. While hospitals are far from the open-air sanatoriums Brian described, it is our hope that hospitals will position themselves to become "palaces for the people."[47]

In this final chapter we have identified specific strategies for moving in this direction and emphasized the contextual nature of this work. Progress will be uneven and often protracted. Some changes may occur organically, as norms evolve alongside new ways of thinking about population health, political pressures to do community-oriented work, and the introduction of new policy. Policies, however, require both institutional and cultural change, as well as effective oversight and enforcement levers, if they are to compel action.[48]

Of course, underlying these forces, at least on some level if maximal effectiveness is the goal, must be a broad grassroots push by residents, especially via the associations we have described here. Local, state, and federal representatives of hospital communities should push for these changes as well. We have noted, for example, that while state government should push hospitals to take community benefit more seriously, the federal government is likely to be less sensitive to well-organized local and state stakeholder advocacy organizations, especially state hospital associations and other industry groups, that may resist efforts to push hospitals to invest more in communities.

Cosgrove's comments, in the quote discussed earlier in this chapter, capture another important aspect of the ongoing changes affecting hospitals and medical centers. He tacitly acknowledged that healthcare institutions might rightfully be subjected to new expectations and regulations, but also demanded that hospitals not be singled out. A key point of this book, however, is precisely that hospitals are singular institutions. They are unique *anchor* institutions, as we have shown, whose missions differ in key ways from the missions of not only other nonprofit and public entities, but also educational institutions and corporations. The data we have brought to bear in this book clarify that community expectations reflect these essential differences.

Persistent and fast-paced changes in medicine and the larger systems encompassing medicine will continue to apply pressure on healthcare institutions in both predictable and unpredictable ways. This book has cataloged some of the extant dynamics in communities near urban hospitals, and has also drawn out hidden yet pervasive dynamics to provide social scientists with scholarly tools for understanding these spaces in the future.

It is both inadvisable and increasingly untenable to operate in a presentist mode while doing community-oriented work. Indeed, the work ahead must reckon with the past even as it looks to the future. Wrestling with the deeper histories through which communities process their own experiences, not only with medicine, but with healthcare-institutions-*as*-urban-institutions, will be a central component of twenty-first-century community health and well-being. As we have shown, hospitals with longer histories often have much to answer for, especially with respect to their deeply racialized histories. Yet newer hospitals, gaining footholds in dynamic urban communities that provide opportunities for new first impressions and possibilities for collaboration, often fare no better. There is a lack of success in both contexts, we argue, because hospitals both old and new must fundamentally rethink the very meaning of being a hospital in the twenty-first century.

We described initial efforts some hospitals have made to address past wrongs, though they are unlikely to be sufficient. Relationship-mending and relationship-building are critical to fostering the types of cross-sector and community-engaged partnerships necessary to truly improve health outcomes in the areas near major urban hospitals. We also provided glimpses of the inspiring work some hospitals are engaging in based on a genuine interest in improving health outcomes, reducing disparities, and simply being a better neighbor. Yet as hospitals envision their futures within their communities, they must juxtapose and examine historical and present perspectives in a way that guides long-term planning, from mission to space, from practices within hospital walls to practices well outside those walls.

These challenges are daunting. The future positioning of healthcare institutions within cities is just as complicated as the multifaceted histories, interests, expectations, and contexts that influenced hospitals as they developed into major urban institutions.

Acknowledgments

The idea of "community" takes pride of place in this book, and so it is important for us to recognize and thank the people who helped with this project, across many years, and many miles. Writing a book is a collective effort and, beyond the names on the front cover, an indispensable community of researchers, readers, and supporters made this text possible.

First, we would like to thank our fantastic teams of graduate and undergraduate student researchers, who helped us with myriad small and large tasks: Noah Barr, Julia Flint, Jory Gomes, Rachel Kamat, Jessica Roth, Madi Shtrahman, Abigail Stephens, and Michael Wright from Ohio University; and Rachel Ayotte, Sam Cadwell, Anna Calamis, Tom Corcoran, Jennifer Garfield-Abrams, Peter Kent-Stoll, Katie Reynolds, Taro Tsujimoto, and Choonhee Woo from the University of Massachusetts Amherst. An extra shout-out to the student researchers who joined us on interviews and research visits: Jennifer at UMass Amherst and Mike, Rachel, and Jessica at Ohio University.

We also thank a group of readers and interlocutors, including Andrew Deener, Teresa Gonzales, Patrick Inglis, Kelly Kelleher, Ivan Kuzyk (author of *A Hartford Primer & Field Guide*), Joan Maya Mazelis, Daniel Menchik, Kelly Nottingham, Liz Polizzi, Jennifer Reich, and the faculty and graduate students of the Department of Landscape Architecture and Regional Planning at UMass Amherst. Access to archival records was provided by the staff at the University of Colorado Strauss Health Sciences Library, Anschutz Medical Campus, and the Health Science Libraries & Hamilton Archives at Hartford Hospital.

Support staff on our respective campuses also deserve our gratitude: Maureen McCann and Cassie Tritipo, Administrative Specialists, who provided invaluable support at Ohio University's Dublin and Athens campuses, respectively, and Karen Mason at the Institute for Social Science Research and Cindy Patten in Sociology at UMass Amherst. The authors have support teams at home as well. Being away from family to do field research can be taxing on families. Dan is grateful for Emily and Zeb's patience and support over the extended course of this research, much of which required travel. Jon is incredibly grateful for the inspiration from his father, Ralph, whose unwavering dedication to his patients and their families at Buffalo's Oishei Children's Hospital inspired much of Jon's thinking in this book, as well as for all the support from Robyn, Ellis, and Yun-sol. Berkeley is grateful to Mark and their late dog, Dublin, who happily joined for research trips to Cleveland, Hartford, and Aurora.

Most important, we want to thank all of our participants, who took time out of their lives to share their stories and communities with us. At times, their experiences in and around urban hospitals were inspiring and hopeful, but often they were painful to recount. We are greatly indebted to many gatekeepers and neighborhood brokers who helped us connect with residents and informants, with special appreciation for Aundra Willis, Rich McClean, and Lee Lazar, each of whom went above and beyond to support this project. We hope our book contributes, even in some small measure, to ongoing efforts to improve health in these neighborhoods and the lives of those who live and work there.

We are grateful for the rock-star duo at the University of Chicago Press who marshaled us through the process with sound advice—our excellent Assistant Editorial Director and Executive Editor, Elizabeth Branch Dyson, and Assistant Editor Mollie McFee—as well as our insightful and generous anonymous reviewers. Thanks are also due to our word wizards, Jennifer Eggerling-Boeck (at Harvest Editing) and Marianne Tatom, who helped make our three voices sound like one on the page.

We are heartbroken that we cannot share this book with some of the key friends and informants we have lost during the multiyear course of this study. Longtime University of Chicago Press Executive Editor Doug Mitchell's early and enthusiastic support made this book possible. Within the communities we studied, Billings Forge Community Works Executive Director Cary Wheaton and Hough community activist Mansfield Frazier were true anchors of their communities. The impact of all three runs throughout this book.

Last, we hope readers will be inspired to visit and support the wonderful communities of Fairfax/Hough, Frog Hollow, and North and South Aurora. These neighborhoods host dynamic local businesses and nonprofits that create the vital fabric of their cities, in obvious and hidden ways. If there is any lesson we have taken from our occasionally vigorous critique of unmet expectations from hospitals, it is that these communities thrive because of the residents who care most about them.

Appendix A: On Methods

To examine our book's central paradox, we widened our scope to the metaphorical bird's-eye view, while still giving voice to the people who live and work at this intersection of hospital and community. This wasn't an easily accessible perspective, even to someone like Anita, one of our interviewees, who was a longtime Clevelander and an urban planner. We asked her about the relationship between local institutions and neighborhoods and she, understandably, took a minute to gather her thoughts: "I barely got [a sense of it] myself, you know? I wouldn't have . . . Okay. So, hold on. Let me think about this for a second. But the neighborhoods are going to be represented in the work, right? The neighborhoods and the institutions. So . . . I have to think about that." For a greater sense of this large puzzle, we matched data provided by people like Anita with the viewpoints of 205 other interviewees. Our respondents were from a wide range of positions from our three cities, and the historical and present conditions of the neighborhoods surrounding hospitals and the dynamics within them.

This approach sits at the intersection of three fields of study: community (including community health) studies, urban and health policy, and studies of urban institutions. From our recruitment of interviewees through the presentation of data to the final editing of the manuscript, our guiding premise has been to put the perspectives of the powerful in conversation with the lived histories and present of the people in the communities around hospitals. And so, although it was not present at the start of the project, as we collected data we grew inspired by recent calls for a greater embrace of the work of W. E. B. Du Bois, while also thinking about how we can gain greater insight into these powerful urban institutions.

In "The Study of Negro Problems"—an essay from 1898 that Itzigshon and Brown suggest serves as a kind of methodological appendix to the classic community study, *The Philadelphia Negro*—Du Bois proposed four components for studying urban communities: a "historical study" of place, "statistical investigation," "anthropological measurement" of race, and "sociological interpretation."[1] The last was the most valuable to Du Bois, as it was "the arrangement and interpretation of historical and statistical matter in the light of the experience of other[s]," which includes the lived perspectives of African Americans. In summary, Itzigshon and Brown detailed how a "Du Boisian Methodology" should meet five criteria: contextualization, relationality, historicity, subaltern standpoint, and theorizing from lived experience.

This method comported with our own multi-perspectival approach to understanding this vast landscape of people and places. *The City and the Hospital* is attuned to all five facets outlined above. First, chapter 1 provides the local and global articulations of power. Second, we were interested in examining the interrelationship between hospitals and urban communities through three different research sites in order to make relational comparisons across cases, but also the perspectives from inside and outside these institutions. Third, chapter 2 is a careful examination of the understanding of the history of the local and the historical nature of the issues at hand. Fourth, in all chapters, *The City and the Hospital* acknowledges that there is a multitude of perspectives from the peripheries and margins. And last, throughout this book we took care to not elevate the voices of the privileged over those with less power and, instead, placed perspectives in greater conversation.

On this last point, our holistic approach to the community/hospital relationship necessitated inclusion of those who have what scholars would call "relative power."[2] What we mean by relative power is that many of our interviewees who served as healthcare administrators and government officials were rarely at the very top of the bureaucracy or part of an economic "super class,"[3] although we interviewed people in city hall, those who sat at the board of directors level, and several people who either were vice presidents at the time of our interview or were in positions of that nature. (And occasionally, we drew upon publicly available interviews to capture the perspectives of those in top leadership roles.) These interviewees certainly had some disproportionate power over the conditions of these neighborhoods. Excluding the viewpoints of these decision-makers would only lend a partial view to this important urban dynamic.

Our multi-perspectival approach complements knowledge and understanding from different positions. The meanings and understandings from all people in this relationship are bound to historical events, movements, traumas, and changes, all of which are parts of an ongoing conversation between hospitals and their communities. We were mindful that local and neighbor-hood histories are essential guides, particularly as they often emanate from communities reeling from decades of marginalization and disinvestment. This is as true of our understanding of the situations within these cities, as it is of the likelihood that any one policy recommendation will be sufficient to address the needs we identify.

Before moving on to specific methodological considerations, we wanted to note that, like many scholars, the COVID-19 pandemic negatively impacted our research agenda. Our data collection was largely complete at the start of 2019, but the pandemic prevented additional site visits and impeded our planned analysis and publication schedules. And, as with any long-term project, there were transitions we had to contend with as we prepared this manuscript for publication. Many of our respondents moved on from the professional posi-tions in which we first encountered them and, tragically, in two cases, our re-spondents passed away: Cary Wheaton and Mansfield Frazier were passionate advocates for their communities, in Hartford and Cleveland, respectively. Their contributions to this book are key to our understanding of their communities, and we benefited greatly from our conversations with them.

Field Site Selection

We selected three sites in order to have what Andrew Deener called "strategic variation":[4] the University of Colorado Hospital (and the Anschutz campus on which it is located), the Cleveland Clinic, and Hartford Hospital provided an excellent set of variables for examination and reflection, in terms of size, status, and geographic region.

Readers should, of course, take reasonable caution when attempting to gen-eralize in any study.[5] However, our three cases provided great data for valuable comparisons.[6] There were clear commonalities, of course, and we highlighted them; but we continually cautioned ourselves against making broad or general claims. There are thousands of hospitals in the U.S., and, as we have argued, attending to the particular and changing roles of these institutions is vital for improving population health outcomes and addressing disparities. Still, we are confident these sites provided us with tools for thinking analytically about the conditions present on other campuses and in different communities.

Interviewees

We formally interviewed 206 people across the three sites (82 in Aurora, 59 in Cleveland, 65 in Hartford) between October 2016 and June 2018. As we explained above, interviewees were from a wide range of positions in and around our three hospital sites and their communities, including administrators and employees, community-based organization leaders, real estate brokers, local business owners, foundation presidents, food activists, police, university campus administrators, government representatives, and everyday folks who live near each medical institution. Our approach was akin to "theoretical sampling":[7] we cast a wide net to capture an array of perspectives, but we also made several course corrections when we realized that we were missing a key perspective. Informal conversations with people at each site—at hotels, restaurants, and elsewhere—helped round out our total understanding of important issues within the community, and helped identify additional informants.

Overall, hospital administrators and healthcare professionals appeared eager to talk with us at length. However, gaining access to administrators and other professionals within hospital systems sometimes required significant effort. The Clinic and Anschutz campus administrators gave us highly curated tours of their facilities, for example, and our initial interviews were quarterbacked by the Clinic's top public relations person. At Hartford Hospital, for example, they directed us to an emeritus professor, and set up a very nice conference room in which to conduct the interview. At all three sites, we were directed to "community-facing" VPs and staffers. These were decidedly not the total of our interviews with hospital employees, however, as we could also talk with others whom we connected with outside of official channels, some of whom requested (and were granted) anonymity. From these initial interviews we used what Jennifer Reich, in her study of anti-vaccine communities, called an "inconvenience sample": we spent significant energy to reach additional and more elusive administrators and staffers, to gain greater and occasionally diverse insight, and we can characterize these efforts as marginally successful.[8]

We were creative in our efforts to interview residents. We sought various ways to engage individuals in public spaces near hospital facilities. For example, we set up a table at a farmers market at Billings Forge, only a few blocks from Hartford Hospital. Two of our research assistants visited a church in Aurora and, with the help of a pastor, interviewed several parishioners after the service. Nonprofit leaders in all communities were gracious in their willingness to connect us with residents in their networks. And for others, we used publicly available contact information to reach out to nonprofit workers, healthcare providers, and academics. In all cases, as part of a snowball sampling strategy,[9] our final interview question was a request for names for additional people to contact.

TABLE A.1. Primary organizational and relational identity across three sites

Position	Example titles	Aurora	Cleveland	Hartford	#
Academics	Deans, Historians, Academic administrators, Professors	9	8	1	18
City government	Mayors, City planners, Superintendents of schools	10	4	7	21
Community leaders	Program directors, Activists, Cultural institution directors	1	4	3	8
Community nonprofit workers	Directors, Community development officers	5	9	8	22
Faith-based nonprofits	Pastors	4	2	2	8
Foundations	Presidents, Vice presidents, Grants officers	1	4	3	8
Health-based nonprofits	Case workers, Community mental health workers, Directors, Public health nutritionists	6	3	11	20
Hospital administrators	Board of directors, Regional vice presidents, Vice presidents for health affairs	3	7	8	18
Hospital employees	Campus safety officers, Physicians, Human resource officers	4	5	1	10
Local business owners	Restaurant proprietors	1	2	-	3
Media	Journalists, Bloggers	-	1	1	2
Residents	N/A	38	10	20	68
Totals		82	59	65	206

Table A.1 summarizes the kinds of ties our respondents held either before or during our interviews. Importantly, while 69 respondents are classified as "residents," because of the specific context in which we interviewed, many of our interviewees (health professionals, advocates and activists, business owners) identified themselves as residents besides their official professional positions. These 69 respondents were not interviewed based on their organizational relationship, but upon their residency proximate to the hospitals, and are identified in the table above.

When it was important context for their perspectives, we identified the geographic and organizational relationships of the respondents (e.g., "When we visited the HHC offices, a block and a half from Hartford Hospital, we interviewed Grace Damio, Director of Research and Service Initiatives").

Understandably, some respondents changed roles, and we tried to signify that change to the best of our abilities without compromising readability (e.g., Kristen Morris, "former Chief Government and Community Relations Officer, Cleveland Clinic").

We did not explicitly inquire about or code respondents' race and gender in our interviews. In aggregate, we determined a best guess for ensuring broad and adequate overall representation and diversity of perspectives among our interviewees across all three locations. We believe we achieved these goals. Regarding race, we were careful to interview respondents from these racially segregated communities, and almost three-quarters of our respondent pool were non-white. Regarding gender, 121 were women and 85 were men ($n = 206$).

Interviewing

Although this book couldn't allow for a rich description of the settings of each of our interviews, we met with our respondents in just about every type of location—in and around hospitals—as could be expected. A total of 18 were in interviewees' residences, 80 were in formal settings (e.g., hospital campuses, clinics, nonprofit offices, churches, community centers), 7 were in government offices, and the rest were in a variety of other venues (e.g., farmers market, hotel lobby, restaurants, and cafés). A total of 66 interviews were conducted via phone. We secured IRB approval from Ohio University and the University of Massachusetts Amherst.

Pilot interviews, publicly available quantitative data, and archival data informed our interview questionnaire. One or two of the researchers, sometimes with the help of research assistants, conducted most of these interviews. In a handful of instances, we had research assistants in Aurora and Cleveland interview with residents in order to maximize time on-site.

We offered incentives to residents, not hospital administrators and staff— thanks to an Ohio University grant. Of the 84 residents to whom we offered incentives, 12 either declined or did not respond to multiple attempts to plan to send them an incentive.

Once we conducted and transcribed all our interviews, we coded the data using established techniques that ensured we were interpreting the data in similar ways. Specifically, we established 248 codes, applying them line-by-line to all interview transcripts. At least two authors coded each interview, and we met regularly to discuss our individual approaches to the application of emerging thematic codes and, sometimes, to merge duplicative codes. These 248 codes capture a wide range of themes, from well-known categories within the social determinants of health to concepts more commonly associated with political science and sociology (e.g., "History of Hospital," "Parking and Traffic," "Healthcare Access," "Disparities," "Schools," and "Partnerships"). Based on our approach to data collection, the breadth of these categories (which, again, arose from the interviewees themselves) is testament to how much there remains to learn from people involved in hospital/community relationships, as well as through a rich, theoretically open-minded approach to the question itself.

Throughout the process, we matched our qualitative interviews with a range of supporting evidence—some of which is presented in tables, charts, and appendixes—to bolster our findings: archival data from hospital libraries, news reports and websites, and census tract demographic information on health outcomes and disparities.

On Using Pseudonyms

It is common practice for qualitative researchers to grant anonymity to their respondents in order to provide greater freedom to speak. Such a practice is important, and respondents were well aware that leaders in the hospitals and in their communities could read their responses. This was particularly true for people who worked in nonprofits that had existing relationships with hospitals, or that aspired to have a relationship with their hospital.

As we might expect, sometimes residents who signaled they had something critical to say about their hospital would hesitate. Residents often prefaced their comments with an appreciation of their hospital's status or ranking, or their excellent clinical care, even if they themselves didn't directly benefit from it. Residents would, however, exhibit some unease if they were to pivot to say anything more negative. Some residents would, for example, joke that they better not say something negative in case they have a heart attack and need care. Others tempered their concerns, often through guarded and even euphemistic language, or broadly wishing for solutions to address health disparities. For us, these interactions were constant reminders that hospitals exert considerable power and the importance of anonymizing our residents.

There are arguments against the practice of using pseudonyms, however, particularly when interviewing those who hold powerful positions.[10] Interviewees, we felt, should have the right to waive their anonymity, and we respected their choice in all cases. And so, before our interviews, we gave respondents the opportunity to waive their anonymity, and 76 did so. The balance of our interviews are therefore presented anonymously. As expected, most of the 76 who waived anonymity were respondents who were in various positions of power and felt comfortable lending their real names to their statements. With interviewees who were residents and who were not being asked about their institutional affiliations, we deidentified them (e.g., "A resident told us . . ."). This was partially to protect the respondents, but also because identifying respondents who were quoted only once or twice would have created far too many individual names for readers.

In cases when we used real names, we reached out to each interviewee at the final draft stage to notify them not only of what quotes we planned on using in the book, but the context within which we were doing so. This allowed our respondents the opportunity to update and adjust their comments to better match any changing conditions or additional reflections. For the researchers, this also allowed us the opportunity to vouchsafe that we did, in fact, get the data and our analysis correct. One of the authors (Wynn) used this method in prior publications.[11]

Funding

We received funding for certain aspects of the research for this book. Skinner and Franz received a $9,002 award through Ohio University's Baker Award Fund, which supported the bulk of travel and incentives for interviewees. They also received smaller awards through the Ohio University Honors Tutorial College Research Apprentice program, the Program to Aid Career Exploration, and the Heritage College of Osteopathic Medicine Office of Research and Grants, Research and Scholarly Advancement Fellowship. From the University of Massachusetts Amherst, professional development funds paid for travel and qualitative data software, and for graduate student research assistants.

The Research Team

As scholars and mentors, we were eager to bring graduate and undergraduate students into the research process. Graduate students joined us on interviews and research visits, and helped collect contact information, archival data, and many other support activities, including the organization of these institutions' complex histories. All students with access to the data received CITI training and IRB approval. Sometimes students actively took part in interviews. Along the way, these students learned how to navigate a semi-structured interview guide, ensure ethical research practices, and handle technical aspects of recording and compliant storage. As noted, internal grants made this mentoring experience possible, culminating in two of the students conducting group interviews in Cleveland and Aurora. All students are thanked in the acknowledgments.

Costs and Benefits

Every research approach has its opportunities and trade-offs. Because we conducted research in three different sites, we could not track as closely as we might have developments—especially infrastructural developments—taking place on the campus over the years in which we were conducting data analysis and drafting the manuscript. The COVID-19 pandemic added a layer of distance between data collection and an intimate understanding of recent developments in these three cities, though Skinner and Franz's proximity to Cleveland, and Wynn's proximity to Hartford, helped close this gap somewhat. In the end, we feel that the benefits of our approach far outweighed the costs: we gained a multi-sited, multi-perspectival view of the interactions between cities and hospitals. As no study can fully examine the many aspects of community health, taking a highly targeted and limited approach for good reason, the benefits of a wider-scale analysis are on display between the covers of this book. The authors, however, enthusiastically invite future research that attends to more of the interactions and lived experiences in these communities.

Appendix B: Comparative Data

TABLE B.1. Comparative social, economic, and health data for the cases, their cities, and the United States

	National avg	Cleveland Clinic Neighborhood	City avg	University of Colorado Hospital Neighborhood	City avg	Hartford Hospital Neighborhood	City avg
Prevalence							
High blood pressure	30.51	**46.9***†	40.7	**28.6***	26.9	**31.9**†	34.8
Cancer	5.5	**6.1***†	5.7	**4.5**	5.1	**4.0**	4.4
Asthma	9.7	**12.5***†	11.8	**9.9***†	9.2	**11.7**†	12.5
Heart disease	5.81	**10.2***†	8.4	**5.7***	4.7	**6.1**†	6.1
COPD	6.32	**11.5***†	10.5	**6***	5.1	**6.7**†	7.0
Smoking	18.1	**28.3**†	29.3	**22.8***†	18.6	**20.1**†	20.6
Diabetes	10.81	**20.1***†	16.2	**9.5***	7.5	**13.4**†	14.0
High cholesterol	34.59	**36.8***†	36.1	**33.3***	31.3	**35.7**†	35.8
Chronic kidney disease	2.97	**5.2***†	4.2	**3.1***†	2.6	**3.4**†	3.4
Poor mental health	13.11	**16.7***†	16.5	**14.3***†	12.1	**15.9***†	15.7
Obesity	30.09	**41***†	39.2	**30.8***†	25.5	**34.21**†	35.7
Stroke	3.23	**7.4***†	5.5	**3.4***†	2.7	**3.5**†	3.8
Prevention							
Mammogram	79.19	**80.6***†	78.2	**72.1**	73.3	**83.7**†	84.5
Routine checkup	69.41	**78.8***†	75.5	**57.7**	58.7	**71.5**†	74.2
Cholesterol screening	72.63	**67.2**	69.4	**63.3**	71.7	**65.4**	68.6
Colorectal cancer screening	61.79	**53.5**	53.6	**52.2**	60.2	**53.5**	59.3

continues

	National avg	Cleveland Clinic Neighborhood	City avg	University of Colorado Hospital Neighborhood	City avg	Hartford Hospital Neighborhood	City avg
Social & economic factors							
Unemployment	3.7	21*†	6.9	8.8*†	2.9	16.3*†	5.1
No health insurance	9.5	11.7*†	8.8	28.1*†	12.5	12.1*†	10.1
Poverty	12.4	50.11*†	32.7	26.8*†	10.7	40.4*†	28.1
Demographics							
White	72.7	22.4	40.0	22.4	60.4	19.1	31.3
Black/African American	12.7	67.6*†	48.8	16.3†	16.5	18.1†	37.7
Two or more races	3.2	1.9	4.4	2.2	5.2	2.1	6.4
Hispanic/Latino	17.8	1.9	11.9	51.6*†	28.6	55.3*†	44.3

*higher than city average
†higher than national average

Source: Social & economic factors and Demographic data come from the U.S. Census Bureau. All other data come from the 500 Cities Project. National data from 500 Cities represent the 500 City averages.

Appendix C: Hospital-Identified Needs and Programs

TABLE C.1. Hospital-identified needs and programs developed in community health needs assessments and implementation strategies

Hospital-identified needs	Selected examples of corresponding hospital programs
Cleveland Clinic (2019)	
Access to affordable healthcare	Provide parking vouchers to Emergency Department patients on campuses where parking fees are assessed
Addiction and mental health	Collect unused medications through community-based drop boxes and a collection service
Chronic disease prevention and management	Provide free physical exams, flu shots, exercise courses, health education, cooking classes, and tobacco cessation programs for the surrounding communities at the Cleveland Clinic Langston Hughes Community Health and Education Center in Fairfax
Infant mortality	Outreach events like Community Baby Showers provide health information to families in specific high-risk geographical areas and encourage enrollment in supportive evidence-based programs
Medical research and health professions education	Through the Physician Diversity Scholars Program, build a diverse healthcare workforce in partnership with the Ohio University Heritage College of Osteopathic Medicine
Socioeconomic concerns	Implement a system-wide social determinants screening tool for patients to identify needs such as alcohol abuse, depression, financial strain, food insecurity, intimate partner violence, and stress
Hartford Hospital (2021)	
Social determinants of health	On Site Food Resource Center: Food Pantry in partnership with Foodshare to address food insecurity among patients, their families and staff
Access to care	Community Care Team referrals and Case Management follow-up for interdisciplinary care teams and community linkages to address medical concerns as well as social needs via partnership with Univ. of St. Joseph's Nursing Program area and social service providers

continues

TABLE C.1. (*continued*)

Hospital-identified needs	Selected examples of corresponding hospital programs
Mental health	The Institute of Health, a division of Hartford Hospital, conducted free Mental Health First Aid Trainings for the public
Obesity/physical activity	The Hartford HealthCare Program was developed in partnership with Wholesome Wave and two clinics affiliated with Hartford Hospital, the Hartford Diabetes Lifecare Clinic, and the Adult Primary Care Clinic
Substance abuse	Implement recovery coach model in the ED

University of Colorado–Anschutz Campus (2021)

Access to specialty care	DAWN Clinic interdisciplinary student-run free clinic serving uninsured patients from the Aurora community—Provide sponsorship of technical support for EPIC platform. Perform processing of lab specimens for DAWN patients
Mental health/substance abuse	Assist pregnant patients with treatment of addiction and with connecting to addiction treatment options
Social determinants of health	Provide support for the hire-local program focused on employment of residents from zip codes surrounding Anschutz Medical Campus. Provide support for learn-local program focused on preparing residents for careers in healthcare fields
Cardiovascular health	Provide community outreach including lectures and e-communication on topics that focus on stroke and cardiovascular disease prevention
Obesity	Provide program allowing community-based primary care physicians and patients to consult with UCHealth diabetes specialists through technology

Sources: Cleveland Clinic 2019; Hartford HealthCare 2018; Hartford HealthCare 2021; UCHealth 2019a; UCHealth 2019b.

Notes

Introduction

1. Verderber 2010: vi.

2. Consistent with IRB guidelines, we offered interviewees the option to remain anonymous or to use their real names. For local residents, we used pseudonyms in all cases. Interviewees who chose to use their real names are generally identified by both first and last name. In addition, we have attempted to make it clear, without compromising readability, which names are pseudonyms and which are not. See Appendix A. Note, as well, that while many of our interviewees hold a range of credentials and degrees, the style employed in this book does not include such information within the text. Instead, we identify interviewees by their positions and (where applicable) institutional affiliations. This decision has the added benefit of ensuring that those interviewees who opted to remain anonymous are described in a manner similar to those who are identified, as well as further protecting the identities of our anonymous interviewees.

3. See HRSA's "MUA find" application at https://data.hrsa.gov/tools/shortage-area/mua-find.

4. Health Resources and Services Administration, n.d. "Medically underserved" is a federal designation indicating that too few primary care services are available, which serves as a basis for the establishment of community health centers and other institutions in those areas. Medically underserved areas are closely related—but legally distinct from—Health Professional Shortage Areas, which denote a shortage of a wider range of healthcare professionals and are tied to federal efforts to incentivize emerging health professionals to practice in high-need areas. For our purposes, both designations are especially concerning when considered in relation to the presence of elite medical institutions within those urban communities where limited access to educational opportunities, quality employment, functional public services, and healthy food outlets further degrade health status.

5. Koh et al. 2020.

6. Unless otherwise noted, "residents" refers to individuals living near hospitals, not medical trainees within hospitals.

7. See van Ham and Manley 2012.

8. Sampson 2019.

9. Graham, Ostrowski, and Sabina 2015.

10. Sharkey 2013.

11. MacDorman and Declercq 2019; Centers for Disease Control and Prevention 2020.

12. Schumacher and Wedenoja 2022.

13. According to the American Hospital Association 2022. The remainder of American hospitals are federal (207), nonfederal psychiatric hospitals (635), and 112 classified as "others," which include units within prisons or schools.

14. As Alexander (2021) showed, the "operating surpluses" of nonprofit hospitals are closer to for-profit hospitals than widely recognized. In addition, studies demonstrate that for-profit hospitals often invest in community health improvement at similar levels as nonprofits, based on explicit charitable requirements. See also Franz, Choyke, et al. 2021.

15. Institutions, broadly, can be considered the repositories of a community's enduring values, beliefs, symbols, and practices, while, at the periphery, are the more mundane practices of the everyday (Shils 1975).

16. Urban universities historically distanced themselves from their communities physically (e.g., gates), socially (e.g., providing education primarily to outsiders rather than local communities), and symbolically (e.g., Columbia's efforts to rebrand their neighborhood as "Morningside Heights" rather than "Harlem") (see Baldwin 2021).

17. Baldwin 2021.

18. Wiley 2019.

19. Medical City Healthcare, n.d. Medical City Healthcare is part of HCA HealthCare.

20. See Bartik and Erickcek 2008.

21. See Marwell and McQuarrie 2013.

22. See Marwell and McQuarrie 2013.

23. See, for example, Minkler 2012; Murphy 2014; Freidson 1963; Rosenberg 1987; Shortell, Gillies, and Devers 1995; Sloan 1980; Starr 1982; Wilson 1963.

24. Sampson's (2012) massive and lauded *Great American City* omits hospitals altogether, as do Wilson's *The Truly Disadvantaged* (1987), Small's *Villa Victoria* (2004), and Sharkey's *Stuck in Place* (2013). Wacquant's *Urban Outcasts* (2008) mentions that hospital closings contribute to the "advanced marginalization" of urban residents, and Goffman's *On the Run* (2014) offers ethnographic evidence for the reasons that marginalized groups avoid hospitals. Massey and Denton's *American Apartheid* (1998: 3, 55), Rhomberg's *No There* (2007: 36, 193), Pattillo's *Black on the Block* (2007: 219), and Auyero and Berti's *In Harm's Way* (2015: 62, 92) mention hospitals only in passing.

25. Major events such as hospital relocation and expansion have disrupted community spaces and have contributed to division in urban communities (Logan and Molotch 2007).

26. Rosenbaum 2013.

27. Andrulis 2006: 85.

28. Nassery et al. 2015.

29. For additional information on and images of Clinic facilities, including the VIP rooms, see Naramore et al., n.d.

30. Klinenberg 2018.

31. Kleinman 2015.

32. Skinner, Gardner, and Kelleher 2016.

33. See, e.g., Dubb, McKinley, and Howard 2013.

34. Goodson and Vassar 2011; Park, Lee, and Chen 2012; Clarke et al. 2014.

35. The title of our book is a loose reference to China Miéville's dystopian novel *The City & the City*, in which two different city-states occupy the same geographic area but are administratively and culturally very different—so distinct that residents of one city don't explicitly acknowledge the existence and presence of the residents of the other city.

Chapter One

1. Prakash and Johnny 2015.
2. Artiga and Hinton 2018.
3. Helmuth 2013.
4. Himmelstein and Woolhandler 2016.
5. U.S. Department of Health and Human Services, n.d.; Marmot and Wilkinson 2005.
6. Gaskin et al. 2014.
7. Krieger et al. 2010.
8. Henderson et al. 2016.
9. Bailey et al. 2017; Feagin and Bennefield 2014; Phelan and Link 2015.
10. Gaskin et al. 2014; Kotecki et al. 2019.
11. Kershaw et al. 2017.
12. Geronimus et al. 2001.
13. Hunt, Tran, and Whitman 2015.
14. NYU Langone Health 2022.
15. Verghese 2012. See, e.g., Kao 2001.
16. Begun et al. 2018.
17. Skinner et al. 2018.
18. Zeuli 2015; Punski 2018.
19. See Baltimore City Health Department 2017.
20. Chicago Health Atlas, https://www.chicagohealthatlas.org.
21. On the different access points in such communities, see Hussein, Diez Roux, and Field 2016.
22. The fact that many of these communities remain underserved suggests that many Americans engage in what Danielle Raudenbush (2020) eloquently called "health care off the books," or the use of informal networks and strategies by underserved populations in an attempt to address health problems outside traditional healthcare services, rather than using elite neighborhood institutions.
23. Rosner 1982; Starr 1982; Stevens 1989.
24. Kisacky 2017.
25. See Rosenberg 1987; Thompson and Goldin 1975.
26. Largent 2018.
27. Largent 2018.
28. Starr 1982.
29. Centers for Medicare and Medicaid Services 2021.
30. Gold 2012.
31. Our three hospitals are in states that availed themselves of the federal funds linked to expanding their Medicaid programs. Connecticut, which was the first state in the country to expand, made the change in 2010, with Colorado expanding in 2013 and Ohio in 2014.
32. Catholic Health Association of the United States 2009.
33. A 2020 Government Accountability Office report found that the "IRS does not have authority to specify activities hospitals must undertake and makes determinations based on facts and circumstances," and that "this lack of clarity makes IRS's oversight challenging. Congress could help by adding specificity to the Internal Revenue Code." Further, "according to IRS officials, hospitals with little to no community benefit expenses would indicate potential

noncompliance. However, IRS was unable to provide evidence that it conducts reviews related to hospitals' community benefits because it does not have codes to track such audits." https://www.gao.gov/products/gao-20-679.

34. Internal Revenue Service 2014.

35. Starr 1982.

36. Kisacky 2017; Reynolds 1997.

37. Quadagno 2000.

38. Rothstein 2017; Greene, Blustein, and Weitzman 2006. Additional institutional policies that may challenge trust and limit access include requiring proof of legal residence for medical services, collaborating with immigration enforcement offices, or simply not attending to pervasive bias within employee ranks.

39. Rubin, Singh, and Young 2015, citing Rev. Rul. 56–185, 1956–1 C.B. 202, modified Rev. Rul. 69–545, 1969–2 C.B.117. On charity care, see Frank and Salkever 1991.

40. See Internal Revenue Service 1969.

41. Examining the community benefit spending of tax-exempt hospitals, Young et al. (2013) found that only 5.3 percent of expenditures were for community health improvement, and over 85 percent were for charity care and other patient care services.

42. Internal Revenue Service, n.d.

43. These dynamics persisted well past the 1970s. In the early 1990s, the Board of Trustees of Hartford's Trinity College, located just south of Frog Hollow, considered leaving downtown in the early 1990s (Sullivan and Trostle 2004).

44. The legal foundations of housing in the U.S. have created the conditions for abuses of all sorts. Langston Hughes wrote in his autobiography that in 1910s Cleveland, "Landlords could get as much as three times the rent from African Americans that they could get from whites, because so few homes were available to Black families outside a few integrated urban neighborhoods" (Rothstein 2017: 172–73).

45. Illescas 2016.

46. Bohlen 2016.

47. Weber 2018.

48. While the community outcry about potential Base Realignment and Closure (BRAC) closings was intense and politically controversial, empirical evidence suggests that most closures did not result in the mass unemployment and community devastation that opponents feared. See Cowan and Webel 2005: 2.

49. Scruggs 2020.

50. Roberts 2019.

51. See the U.S. Census estimates at https://www.census.gov/library/publications/2021/demo/p60–274.html. For more on why access to care data is important to understanding barriers to health, see County Health Rankings and Roadmaps, "Access to Care," https://www.countyhealthrankings.org/explore-health-rankings/measures-data-sources/county-health-rankings-model/health-factors/clinical-care/access-to-care.

52. Clough 2004: 45–46.

53. Clifton, n.d.

54. Cleveland Restoration Society, n.d.

55. Boyd 2016.

56. The Clinic also established a relationship with Kaiser Permanente, becoming the primary healthcare provider for Kaiser members in the Cleveland area. While this was in some

ways a controversial partnership because it shut out the institutions that had previously served Kaiser members, it led to physicians in the Ohio Permanente Medical Group being given the privilege to practice at Cleveland Clinic hospitals, and allowed Kaiser Permanente to close their hospitals.

57. These affiliations and mergers included Fairview, Lakewood, Marymount, Summa, and Akron, along with purchases such as the Mount Sinai ambulatory building, which became the Beachwood Family Health Center (Clough 2004: 132–33).

58. Plans for the new Heart Center began in the early 2000s, as did the development of the Cleveland Clinic Lerner College of Medicine of Case Western Reserve University.

59. Cleveland Foundation 2014.

60. The Clinic's 2016 Community Health Needs Assessment noted that "Main Campus communities have comparatively unfavorable socioeconomic indicators, particularly in Medically Underserved Areas." Cleveland Clinic 2016: 28.

61. Cleveland Department of Health, n.d.

62. Diamond 2017a.

63. Cuyahoga County Board of Health 2021. U.S. infant mortality data are available at https://data.worldbank.org/indicator/SP.DYN.IMRT.IN?locations=US. Accessed January 15, 2022.

64. Kirby 2017.

65. See United Nations 2019.

66. One mayor told the *Wall Street Journal* that Hartford is "built on a tax base of a suburb," and said that the state must help bail out the city (De Avila 2017).

67. Lazarus 1991: 23; Clouette and Lever 2004: 30.

68. DeBoer 2014.

69. The number of downtown parking spaces has tripled since the 1960s. Plans to redevelop the viaduct to limit these effects stalled in 2019.

70. According to Campbell (2019), "A marsh gives the neighborhood its name, though subsequent generations once claimed that the 'frog' came from the influx of French Canadians who began moving to the hollow in the 1850s to work in the factories."

71. Federal Information Processing Standards, or FIPS, code 5003.

72. Commonwealth Fund 2020.

73. See Hughes et al. 2021; Franz, Parker, et al. 2021.

74. IRS Form 990 and Schedule H data from Communitybenefitinsight.org.

75. Lown Institute Hospitals Index, "Community Benefit."

76. The American Hospital Association believes the Lown Institute's findings "fall short," noting that many additional benefits to communities were not included in their data, and instead refer to findings that for every dollar spent on a tax-exempt hospital, $11 of benefits are returned to the community (Pollack 2021).

77. Atkeson and Higgins 2021.

78. Davidson and Ward 2018.

79. See Martin 2014. Hartford has been the focus of rancorous budgeting debates, with state legislators, especially Republican legislators, frustrated about the need for state monies to help Hartford return to solvency and pay off debts approaching $1 billion. As a result of legislative jockeying between the city and state, threats to cut state monies in other areas, including resources on which the city depends (such as services provided by the Department of Children and Families), have created a budgetary climate in which basic municipal services are continually at risk of being slashed.

Chapter Two

1. Du Bois 1899: 162.

2. According to Hirschman and Reed (2014: 260), these stories are "points of reference" and their trajectories are a "messy, heterogeneous process." Furthermore, "some actions, accidents, decisions, and details are causally much more important than others, in terms of how they shape the future of social life from a certain point in time and space. Some occurrences change the fabric of social reality."

3. These laws were reversed in 2021, protecting and supporting the state's undocumented residents.

4. Jones 2015.

5. *The Sentinel* 2015.

6. Andersen 1995; Freidson 1970; Pescosolido 1992.

7. Geertz (1983: 167).

8. Corburn 2005.

9. Acosta 2020.

10. Though the health professions workforce is becoming more diverse, it remains dominated by white professionals. See U.S. Department of Health and Human Services 2017.

11. Lipsitz 2011: 209. Du Bois, who was encouraged by an editor to delete some of his retelling of history to focus on the present, fantasized about offering the following response: "Dear, dear Jackass! Don't you understand that the past *is* the present; that without what *was*, nothing *is*?" (Du Bois 1965: 80).

12. Subica and Link 2022. These traumas can be specific (e.g., around physical buildings or events) or more diffuse (e.g., the feeling of what a neighborhood was or the loss of a potential future for the community) (see Fentress and Wickham 1992: ix).

13. Komarnisky et al. 2016. Other research has shown how oral histories shed light on barriers to healthcare utilization and help researchers engage locals in the process of cataloging existing assets and addressing needs (Drees 2013; Hernandez et al. 2017).

14. See Gamble 1997.

15. Canada and Carter 2021.

16. Institute of Medicine Committee on Understanding and Eliminating Racial and Ethnic Disparities in Health Care 2003.

17. See O'Reilly 2020; American Hospital Association 2020.

18. Beyond explicit mistreatment, exploitation, and discrimination in clinical spaces, histories of disinvestment and redlining in urban neighborhoods exacerbate mistrust in institutions more broadly. Kevin Nowak, Executive Director of a local nonprofit promoting homeownership in Cleveland, told a local NPR station that "particularly in areas on Cleveland's East Side and in inner-ring suburbs, you see a significant lack-to-no mortgage activity. And many times, those areas also mimic the areas that were redlined areas back in prior decades."

19. Georgetown University 2016.

20. Johns Hopkins Medicine n.d.; Skloot 2010.

21. Prior studies show how hospitals' actions shape public perception of their organizations and of healthcare more generally. Coupled with a history of segregation and exclusion within medical institutions, it is not uncommon for locals to distrust hospitals. Some of this distrust manifests in public attention focused on historical missteps (Quadagno 2000; Arnett et al. 2016; Nandyal et al. 2021).

22. Often women are the ones who hold the memories and are the storytellers of these community memories (see Schoenberg 1980: 263).

23. Goffman 1974; Collins 2004: 32–42.

24. Case Western Reserve University, n.d.

25. Willis-Carrasco, n.d.

26. Andrzejewski and Abbott 1977; *Call and Post* 1982.

27. Chowkwanyun 2018.

28. Donnan 2020.

29. Rice 1979.

30. See Neubeck and Ratcliff 1988: 323.

31. Rojas 2015.

32. Papirno and Rhinelander 1973.

33. Hooker 1974: 3, Papirno 1974; Cruz 1998: 170–72; Singer 2003.

34. Using a community-based approach, the HHC seeks to empower the community and strengthen community voices, building on its role in the community during the 1990s HIV/AIDS epidemic, but also responding to emerging health challenges in the community. By 1982, HHC's formal mission centered on the provision of direct services, including crisis interventions, family counseling, service referrals, and research/advocacy/training programs. In 1984, the group hosted its first citywide health fair, a program that continues to this day.

35. Schensul et al. 1982.

36. Briggs 2002.

37. Calhoun 2012.

38. Weber 2018.

39. Hunter and Robinson 2018.

40. Morse 2015.

41. See Zhou 1993; Brown-Saracino 2009; Wherry 2010; Molotch, Freudenburg, and Paulsen 2000.

42. Greenberg 2000; Hakala, Lemmetyinen, and Gnoth 2010.

43. In 2017, the metro area's transportation system, the Regional Transportation District, opened a station that brings visitors within a 10-minute walk or a short Anschutz shuttle ride to campus. This accessibility, however, does not increase connectivity with Aurora, but rather with Denver and the surrounding areas.

44. Franz, Skinner, and Murphy 2018.

45. Hughes 2016.

46. Glaser 2016.

47. Trickey 2003.

48. Menchik 2021: 107.

49. Hyra 2012; Etienne 2012.

50. Gonzales 2021: 16. See also Armstrong et al. 2006.

51. LaVeist, Isaac, and Williams 2009; LaVeist, Nickerson, and Bowie 2000.

52. Andersen (1995) revised his framework from the 1960s to emphasize the dynamic interactions between variables such as health outcomes and trust as institutions make decisions about future healthcare utilization.

53. Weyeneth 2001.

54. AHRQ 2017.

55. Laurencin 2021.

Chapter Three

1. Rienzi 2013.
2. See Ahmed et al. 2019.
3. Erickson 2013: 2.
4. See Benit-Gbaffou and Katsaura 2014.
5. Sampson 1991.
6. Solomon and Kanter 2018.
7. ICIC 2016.
8. U.S. Bureau of Labor Statistics, https://www.bls.gov. Our cities have different unemployment profiles, though recent figures are hard to generalize due to the COVID-19 pandemic. As of November 2021, the unemployment rates in these cities were as follows: Aurora 4.5 percent (Colorado 5.1 percent), Cleveland 3.7 percent (Ohio, 4.5 percent), and Hartford 4.8 percent (Connecticut 6.0 percent), while the overall U.S. unemployment rate was 4.2 percent. Aurora is slightly more difficult to measure than the others, as it is generally included in the Bureau of Labor Statistics' Denver-Aurora-Lakewood statistical area. Aurora-specific data suggest that the city of Aurora's unemployment rates trend slightly below (that is, better than) national averages. Aurora has benefited from the larger growth patterns in the state of Colorado, which is experiencing an economic boom. Similarly, in Cleveland unemployment levels tended to track those of the state of Ohio (Federal Reserve Bank of Cleveland 2019).
9. Median household income in Aurora, according to 2019 U.S. Census data, is $65,100. See https://www.census.gov/quickfacts/fact/table/auroracitycolorado/INC110219.
10. ICIC 2011.
11. Nelson and Wolf-Powers 2010.
12. Gartland said University Hospitals used to "just hire to hire" but now considers employment a way to "invest dollars locally and very proactively."
13. SINA's founding Executive Director and President, Ivan Backer, examined employment records from the 1980s and confirmed this recollection.
14. "The Mondragon model" was developed by a Catholic priest whose idea of worker-owned collectives spawned dozens of enterprises that mutually supported one another. Candi Clouse, then the Interim Director for the Center for Community Planning and Development Program at Cleveland State University, explained that the Clinic also drew on what she called the "Manchester Bidwell Model" and work being done in Pittsburgh, where the Manchester Bidwell Corporation uses career training for adults, youth-focused arts education, and the promotion of social enterprise to help communities of color thrive. See Evans-Pritchard 2011.
15. Schnoke et al. 2018: 19; Ergungor and Oliver 2013.
16. Grzegorek 2018.
17. The program was funded by numerous campus entities and supported by contributions from the City of Aurora and the Denver Foundation.
18. Anschutz's Campus-Community Partnership launched in 2014 to consolidate hiring efforts across the entire campus and avoid competition between departments.
19. Launched in July 2013, the Aurora Strong Resilience Center provided community support after the July 2012 mass shootings; the group was run by the City of Aurora, Anschutz Wellness Center, Colorado Organization for Victims Assistance, and Aurora Mental Health. The hub partnered with a nonprofit "vocational rehabilitation program," and a nonprofit offering extensive outreach and a range of programming, including employment services, to help residents

with applications and resumes. The center closed in 2019, and its responsibilities were transferred to the 501(c)(3) 7/20 Memorial Foundation.

20. Fairfax Renaissance 2020; Hexter et al. 2017.

21. Cleveland's University Hospitals has a workforce preparedness and promotion program
called "Step Up UH" that empowers a nonprofit called Neighborhood Connection to identify, screen, and assist potential job candidates for UH. The NewBridge Cleveland Center for
Arts & Technology is another nearby workforce training and resource center, funded by the
Greater University Circle Initiative (GUCI). UH's Heidi Gartland noted that "Step Up UH" focused on lowering employee turnover, dropping the rate from 80 percent to 20 percent. She
described her concerns about turnover: "The cost of every time you turn over a position . . .
It's expensive."

22. There are also pre-health education programs conducted through a collaboration of the
Colorado University Office of Inclusion and Outreach and the Colorado Area Health Education
Center, which were established by the U.S. Department of Health and Human Services' Health
Resources and Services Administration to connect university health science centers with local
planning, educational, and clinical resources.

23. Desmond 2016.

24. For an overview of this extensive literature, see Taylor 2018.

25. There are some beautiful buildings in downtown Hartford. While San Francisco has its
Painted Ladies, Hartford's archetypical style is the "Perfect Six": two side-by-side, three-story
housing units found around Frog Hollow and throughout Hartford (Hagaman 2016).

26. Funders include the Cleveland Clinic, Cleveland Foundation, Case Western University,
University Hospitals, and a local senior living facility.

27. See Democracy Collaborative, n.d.

28. Minemeyer 2016.

29. This is a national concern. "Just in time" production is becoming increasingly common,
and the consolidation of global supply chains, much of which capitalizes on cheap and even
forced labor in the production of basic commodities required in many industries, is occurring
in the healthcare industry as well. See Green 2015; King 2020.

30. O'Leary 2020.

31. Lara Ann Frey, Program Manager of Natural Helpers, an Aurora program offering leadership training to residents, called these programs "aspirational." Frey indicated that applicants
were not always underqualified. Sometimes, in fact, they were overqualified, and the challenge
was to match the applicant with a position where their skills could be best utilized. She said the
system needs to have a "creative" human resources staff who can place a potentially valuable
employee who speaks multiple languages and has demonstrated an aptitude to learn.

32. All three major anchors in the Greater University Circle Initiative (i.e., the Clinic, University Hospitals, and Case Western University) reported that 5.7 percent of their employees
hailed from surrounding neighborhoods (Hexter et al. 2017: 29–30).

33. Marks reported that the infrastructure is still in development. In 2016, the Cleveland
Clinic hired six full-time employees through the "Welcome to Fairfax" program. A report stated
that 54 Fairfax residents who were in the program found full-time employment, either with
Clinic vendors or outside the Clinic (Hexter et al. 2017: 30). Cleveland State University and the
Cleveland Foundation found that the Greater University Circle's jobs initiatives (e.g., Step Up
UH, the NewBridge Cleveland Center for Arts & Technology, the Evergreen Cooperatives) gen-
erated 429 new jobs (Hexter et al. 2017: 9).

34. Schnoke et al. 2018: 31. Of the seven University Circle neighborhoods, Hough had the second fewest homes purchased through the program.

35. As of winter 2021, SINA had sold 72 houses via Cityscape homes (a program designed to sell renovated and newly constructed homes to low- and moderate-income first-time buyers), operated four land-banked properties, and managed 15 apartments. Cityscape homes are refurbished and built by Pope Park Zion LLC, a developer established and owned by SINA, which is a noteworthy strategy for neighborhood associations.

36. Some locals have hope for market-based redevelopment of old factory spaces. One site, "Capitol Lofts," offers 112 new condominiums, 20 percent of which have been designated as affordable housing. Since 2015, over 800 new apartments have been built in downtown Hartford, and another 600 are planned (Gosselin 2017).

37. Of the Clinic's procurement, 13 percent was from within Cuyahoga County's suburbs and 77 percent was from outside Cuyahoga County (Schnoke et al. 2018: 14). Comparatively, Case Western expended 16 percent of their procurement in the city in 2017, 10 percent in the Cuyahoga County suburbs, and 74 percent outside the county, while University Hospitals expended 14 percent of their procurement in the city, 24 percent in the Cuyahoga County suburbs, and 61 percent outside the county (Schnoke et al. 2018: 14).

38. Cleveland Clinic 2020a: 50.

39. Marcus McKinney, from Hartford's Trinity Health, said Trinity tried to address supply diversity at a smaller scale by "giving opportunities to minority-owned businesses," but such support often came in the form of logistical partnerships rather than "wholesale purchasing."

40. See Molotch 1976.

41. With the rise of healthcare systems, each of these hospitals not only sought to purchase adjacent real estate, but also aspired to expand across the region, which administrators believed was necessary for the institution to survive. Hartford Hospital, for example, became Hartford Healthcare in 2011, using Hartford as its hub. A community organizer remarked, "Most of Hartford Hospital's recent activity in terms of expansion, et cetera, has been fierce competition in the suburbs."

42. The hospital also partnered with the school district to enable siblings of patients to attend a local school.

43. Clough 2004: 92.

44. Hexter et al. 2017.

45. Diamond 2017a.

46. A second corridor a few blocks to the south, running through the Slavic Village, Kinsman, and Fairfax neighborhoods, which some call the city's "Forgotten Triangle," is the focus of a three-mile, $300 million project aimed at stimulating economic development in high-poverty neighborhoods (Litt 2019).

47. Epstein said the corridor is working on digital and broadband inclusion as well as establishing places for not just economic development but community development.

48. *Sheff v. O'Neill*, 238 Conn. 1, 678 A.2d 1267.

49. The Learning Corridor was funded with monies from the State of Connecticut (e.g., Connecticut Departments of Education, Public Works, and Environmental Protection) and from Hartford Hospital, Connecticut Children's Medical Center, the Institute of Living, Connecticut Public Television and Radio, and Aetna Insurance.

50. Stowe 2000.

51. Stroud empathized with parents whose children must enter a lottery for the chance to attend the schools across the street. She said this was a concern early on, but now "the neighborhood sees the advantage, even if their kids didn't come to the school."

52. This phrasing intentionally echoes Wacquant's (2009) formulation of the state's "left hand" (i.e., education, welfare apparatus) and "right hand" (i.e., policing, carceral system).

53. Although hospitals may contribute positively to urban revitalization through expansion and support of local business, rapid neighborhood development can also spur gentrification and displace residents (Skinner, Donovan-Lyle, and Kelleher 2014; Edgar 2018).

54. To learn more about the data and methods used by the Evictions Lab, see https://evictionlab.org/methods/#section-name.

55. What SINA calls the "seventh phase" of its Cityscape program is a continuation of efforts to refurbish several boarded-up and abandoned multi-unit buildings being used for illegal drug use and distribution-only blocks from Hartford Hospital. See Lurye 2021.

56. Hexter et al. 2017: 39.

57. Schnoke et al. 2018: 34.

58. Vacancy rates around Hartford Hospital were greater than the rates in the city at large. For example, 7 percent fewer residents in Frog Hollow were living in their residence than one year prior. Wheaton pointed to what she characterized as "urban pioneering" along the northern edge of Frog Hollow, on Capitol Avenue (see fig. 1.6 in chapter 1). On the heels of the Great Recession, however, from 2009 to 2018, home values dropped 24.76 percent in five of those seven census tracts, relative to a 13 percent drop overall.

59. Tringer 2017.

60. Others, like Jillian, the former Director of an Aurora arts nonprofit, took a comparative perspective, noting that "housing is not as expensive [in Aurora] as in other parts of Denver." Cost-of-living calculators assessed Denver at about 10 percent more expensive than Aurora for all expenses, but up to 30 percent higher for the cost of purchasing a home.

61. Tringer 2017.

62. Bryson 2019.

63. However, he added that, in his estimation, Hartford's institutions have not been particularly focused on land acquisition.

64. Instead of organizing community land trusts, Hartford's SINA coordinates with other nonprofits to develop land-banked properties, refurbishing foreclosed properties and returning them to the market.

Chapter Four

1. Kleinman 2015.

2. Spiro 1990.

3. Releford, Frencher, and Yancey 2010.

4. Pager, Sun, and Wagner 2021.

5. Stefanowicz, Feldman, and Robinson 2021.

6. Pratt 1991: 34. There is also a corollary in Lao-Montes's (2007: 317) concept of the "Black borderlands" as a "geo-historical field with multiple borders and complex layers." See also Finkler, Hunter, and Iedema 2008.

7. Wilson 2011; Schorch 2013; Leitner 2012; Farrer 2011.

8. See Mayblin et al. 2015. Research in social psychology has shown that reducing tension and prejudice between social groups requires the mediation and minimization of power (Anderson 2011).

9. Hartford HealthCare (n.d.), for example, noted that their social workers are "available to support people managing the physical and emotional stress of illness," indicating that the organization does not view social work as a community asset, but rather a support for their work in clinical medicine.

10. Weiss et al. 2006; Garmon and Chartock 2017; Kaiser Family Foundation 2021; Tarraf, Vega, and González 2014; Gordon 1999; Buchbinder 2017; Mannon 1976; Greenwood-Ericksen and Kocher 2019; Blair, Manheim, and Cowper 2002; Berk and Schur 2001; Goffman 2014; Lara-Millán 2021. Lara-Millán described the links between police and ED nurses in detail, from nurses hurrying treatment to arrestees to police running background checks on people in waiting rooms.

11. Though there is an extensive literature demonstrating this point, see Johnson et al. 2012.

12. See the website of the Joint Commission, https://www.jointcommission.org.

13. In 1871, the hospital established a free clinic, the Hartford Dispensary.

14. These statistics are from Hartford Hospital Nurse Manager Pamela Clark's court testimony requesting funds from the state budget (Connecticut General Assembly 2019).

15. Dawn Clinic 2022.

16. Boulder Strong Resource Center 2021.

17. A Cleveland city planner noted that the Clinic's next-door neighbor, University Hospitals, had a "far more welcoming architecture facing the community" than the Cleveland Clinic.

18. Rosenberg 1987: 286–87.

19. Harder 2021.

20. See Appendix A for more detailed information on how we interviewed people in these positions.

21. At the time of this writing, there were more than 350 job listings for "patient navigators" in New York City alone. Such organizational change is not without precedent. Watkins-Hayes (2009) examined how the roles of welfare caseworkers changed after the passage of the 1996 Personal Responsibility and Work Opportunity Act (which implemented often burdensome work requirements); they found that roles shifted from ensuring recipients were qualified to receive welfare benefits to finding resources for recipients seeking employment, thus transforming caseworkers into "catchall bureaucrats."

22. Mailloux and Halesey 2018.

23. There is hope that vendors will be able to address community concerns. David Portillo, for example, expressed some hope that Anschutz could embody the institution's values in its relationships with vendors.

24. See Flores 2005; Flores et al. 2012; Nápoles 2015.

25. Title VI was reaffirmed in a 1974 Supreme Court ruling (*Lau v. Nichols*) and again by an executive order issued by President Clinton in 2000 (Chen et al. 2007).

26. Centers for Medicare and Medicaid Services, "Translation and Interpretation Services" (n.d.).

27. Juckett and Unger 2014.

28. Although some interviewees used the word "translation" in interviews, the more accurate term is "interpretation," which denotes spoken, real-time language support, rather than translation, which usually denotes a written process. See Allen et al. 2020.

29. DeJesus 2009.

30. Understanding security is also essential when studying the relationships communities have with colleges and universities. Davarian Baldwin (2021) illustrates how university public safety departments often do terrible jobs policing campus crimes (e.g., rape, assault) and instead focus on policing neighboring communities. In an interview, Baldwin told a story that resonates with our data: "In 2006, in Chicago, Damian Turner suffered from a gunshot wound just blocks away from the extremely prosperous U Chicago hospital. But they didn't have Level 1 trauma services. So he had to be transferred eight miles away to another hospital, and on the way, he died. Residents, community activists, and students protested for years, and now there is a Level 1 trauma center at the U Chicago hospital. But that was only because of protests, direct action, and campaigning, and because the optics were just so bad" (Day 2021). In light of the wider political climate around policing, Johns Hopkins reconsidered developing its own security force (Johns Hopkins Hub 2021), and many universities are revisiting the idea of campus police as well (Barajas 2020).

31. Cleveland Clinic, n.d.

32. University of Colorado Anschutz Medical Campus 2021. See also *Security Magazine* 2011.

33. According to McCartney, emergency services and the police force work together closely, with "many" police officers having once been paramedics.

34. Police make their incursions into hospital campuses as well: installing license plate readers in ED parking lots, executing warrants and making arrests in EDs, asking physicians and nurses about patients' injuries and diagnoses to benefit investigations, and interacting with patients before and during hospitalization (Burke and Paradise 2015; Brayne 2014; Song 2021: 2650; Lara-Millán 2014; Baker et al. 2016; Jacoby et al. 2018).

35. Buchheit et al. 2021; Green, McCullough, and Hawley 2018.

36. In addition, a lack of mental health services and overworked urban EDs sometimes make them dangerous (Stone et al. 2012; Foust and Rhee 1993).

37. A professor described how the highways surrounding the campus made it hard for visitors, including residents, to access Anschutz. In the same response, however, he said the hospital campus newsletter boosted a "fear of the neighborhoods" by featuring articles on safety and recommendations for where to park when visiting campus.

38. Armstrong 2020a. The report found that between January 1, 2015, and September 2020, University Circle police forces (e.g., Clinic, University Circle, and University Hospitals police) brought over 8,000 criminal charges and traffic citations against 5,600 people, and that three-fourths of those arrested or ticketed were Black. Almost 90 percent of those who were given trespass orders, and over 90 percent of those charged with misdemeanor possession of marijuana, were Black.

39. Armstrong 2020b.

40. Armstrong 2020b.

41. University of Colorado Anschutz Medical Campus 2021.

42. Cleveland Clinic 2020b.

43. U.S. Department of Education 2016.

44. Metzl and Hansen 2014.

45. Romano 2018; Garran and Rasmussen 2019.

46. The Cleveland Clinic (2021) website states: "Our Executive Inclusion and Racial Equity Council promotes policies to build a culture of diversity, equity and inclusion that is free from the racism, bias, and health disparities that adversely impact patients, caregivers, and

communities. Additionally, we've been working to develop programs, partnerships and hiring practices that are dedicated to helping our communities thrive."

47. Lie et al. 2011; Chae et al. 2012.

48. McQuarrie (2013: 148) outlined three phases: CBOs taking part in contentious politics were subsumed by community development groups in the 1970s; the rise of the community development expert; and a stage of participatory practice that "valorizes collaboration and partnership."

49. See Liou and Stroh 1998; Wacquant and Wilson 1989.

50. Franz et al. 2019.

51. Small described these organizations as "provid[ing] a space for both formal and informal social interaction among neighborhood residents. Rather than pursuing single organizational objectives, these organizations and their actors respond to multiple pressures from heterogeneous sources, such as the state, professional norms, and external agencies aiming to target the poor" (2006: 276; see also Allard and Small 2013). Understanding under-resourced communities also means understanding their embedded organizations and the delivery of services they provide.

52. Oliver 2013; Seim 2020.

53. There are two dominant ways of thinking about emerging organizational ecologies: examining how individuals and agencies serve as boundary spanners or brokers, and examining how individuals and organizations vary in their degree of dependence on institutions for resources (e.g., a decades-old tradition of understanding the relationships across organizations in terms of spanning boundaries) (Steadman 1992; Long, Cunningham, and Braithwaite 2013).

54. CDCs arose in the 1970s and 1980s on the heels of the civil rights movement, at a time of rapid and extensive urban disinvestment as well as dramatic decreases in the federal funding of antipoverty programs. As such, CDCs are often oriented toward addressing the impact of disinvestment and redlining on affordable housing. The funding structure was reorganized as the Community Development Block Grant Act of 1974 (Erickson and Andrews 2011).

55. Cowan et al. 1999; von Hoffman 2013.

56. Cleveland's development history emerged through "community foundations and strategic business organizations, rather than through government" (McQuarrie 2013: 152, 158).

57. For example, community residents will be no less than one-third of membership (McQuarrie 2013) and CDCs are organized around a civic or religious organization. CDCs can receive funding from foundations or municipal, state, and federal grants, or can apply through national community development intermediaries (NCDIs).

58. Richter et al. 2017.

Chapter Five

1. For Fukuyama (1995: 26), trust is an expansive concept, defined as follows: "the expectation that arises within a community of regular, honest, and cooperative behavior, based on commonly shared norms, on the part of other members of that community." See also Robbins 2012; Leblang and Satyanath 2006.

2. It is undeniable that, in a post-Watergate era, Americans still have a "crisis of confidence" in institutions broadly. Low expectations of government and corporations bleed into expectations of other generally respected institutions, including hospitals.

3. John 2021.

4. Mettler 2011.

5. At the level of city government there is often a perception that health is someone else's jurisdiction. A survey of over 100 U.S. mayors found consensus that health is not directly under the purview of municipal governments, but rather is the responsibility of counties, states, and the federal government. Moreover, mayors tended to rank municipal priorities in a way that did not align with what public health tells us are the most effective ways to promote health and reduce disparities (such as messaging campaigns, investments in community health centers, targeted interventions, and the regulation of risk factors). In addition, while "Mayors see obesity and other chronic diseases, opioids, and access to care as the leading health challenges facing their community," they also say their constituents tend to hold them accountable for different priorities, such as traffic accidents (Lusk and Wang 2019).

6. Wyland 2013.

7. See Young and Billings 2020.

8. American Hospital Association 2019.

9. Franz, Skinner, and Murphy 2018; Skinner, Franz, and Kelleher 2018.

10. Cronin and Bolon 2018; Bolon 2005.

11. AAMC 2020.

12. Institute of Medicine 1997.

13. Even locals who were unaware of a hospital's actual fiscal health, legal obligations, and community benefit assessments often had some sense of vast resources that were not being leveraged for community health. As noted in earlier chapters, it is challenging to identify and fully assess the investments hospitals make in community health, despite the ACA's requirement to make that information publicly accessible (Public Health Institute 2017). As required by law, Community Health Needs Assessments are relatively easy to locate on hospital websites; however, more fine-grained financial data are harder to access, especially for residents who stand to benefit the most from the community benefit investments of their hospital. American healthcare, of course, is notoriously opaque, even for nonprofit hospitals (Adams 2021).

14. See Alexander 2021.

15. In this regard, medical institutions are not much different than developments such as sports arenas, business hubs, and warehouses (see MacGillis 2021).

16. Winant 2021.

17. While transportation is a serious issue for patient care and has received a good deal of attention in recent years, including from state Medicaid programs (Musumeci and Rudowitz 2016) and the American Hospital Association (Health Research & Educational Trust 2017), how hospitals affect transportation systems, including traffic itself, has rarely been considered by U.S. researchers. This is not the case in other countries. The British National Health Service (NHS), for example, acknowledged that its carbon footprint is unsustainable. Among other things, the NHS's climate strategy includes a "Long Term Plan commitment to better use technology to make up to 30 million outpatient appointments redundant, sparing patients thousands of unnecessary trips to and from hospital" (National Health Service 2020).

18. Such expectations are often only heightened when catastrophes (e.g., earthquakes, hurricanes, wildfires, and pandemics) befall cities. During such crises, hospitals may take on new meanings for residents. Consider how New Orleanians viewed their hospitals during and after Hurricane Katrina, as sites of both heroism and dysfunction that failed to serve them in fundamental ways (Fink 2013).

19. Franz, Skinner, and Murphy 2018.

20. Somerville et al. 2015.

21. Donor fatigue is another force causing further erosion of expectations, as when an insti-tution insists that it has done its best and provided sufficient support and investment to a com-munity, and determines that the community will never regard its investments as sufficient (re-lating to perceived capacity). For nonprofits and community members seeking to partner with hospitals, the prospect of hospitals adopting these modes of reasoning is alarming. Residents' low expectations are similarly alarming, and a significant roadblock to progress.

Chapter Six

1. Luthi 2019.

2. Sanger-Katz 2019.

3. Recall that the Cleveland Foundation—one of the oldest and most powerful foundations in the country—brought together the Clinic, University Hospitals, and Case Western to form the powerful Greater University Circle Initiative, and sent anchor administrators to Spain to learn about worker-owned collectives. Similarly, the Denver Foundation served as a convener, bringing together Anschutz Medical Campus administrators, provided a small grant to their Community-Campus Partnership to employ a community organizer, and helped Anschutz ad-ministrators travel to Cleveland to learn about "hiring local" programs. Further, the Hartford Foundation for Public Giving did something similar, paying for a community organizer in a role that blossomed into SINA.

4. A study by the Anchor Institutions Funders Group identified five types of activities in which anchors can play especially meaningful roles: convening, fostering collaborations, com-munity development grants, leadership and capacity building, and research (Pease 2017: 7, 12).

5. Milken Institute, n.d.

6. Ross 2014.

7. Health Resources & Services Administration, "Chapter 20: Board Composition," https://bphc.hrsa.gov/programrequirements/compliancemanual/chapter-20.html.

8. See Centers for Medicare and Medicaid Services, "CMS' Value-Based Programs"; Centers for Medicare and Medicaid Services, "Value-Based Purchasing." Despite a great deal of excite-ment among some scholars about this move to "value," it is unclear whether these policies will deliver on their promise (see Crosson 2011). This includes the Centers for Medicare and Med-icaid Services' "shared savings programs" conducted via new institutional models such as the Accountable Care Organizations established by the ACA. Though some have predicted that Accountable Care Organizations are "doomed for failure" (Weil 2012), the broader consensus is that Accountable Care Organizations and other emerging models based on alternative payment systems are essential for moving beyond outdated aspects of the U.S. healthcare system. To push nonprofit healthcare institutions to assume financial risk in a way that forces them to become more open to initiatives that stand to improve population health, shared-savings programs must be integrated into a growing number of institutions.

9. Kocher and Rajkumar 2021.

10. Committee on Accounting for Socioeconomic Status in Medicare Payment Programs 2016.

11. See Rao et al. 2020.

12. Paremoer et al. 2021.

13. Rosenbaum 2013.

14. Bentley et al. 2008; Detrow and Rosenthal 2021.

15. American Academy of Family Physicians 2022.

16. Henderson 2021.

17. Patow et al. 2016.

18. There are examples of church-based programs that engage local histories in the training of lay community health workers to encourage conversations about the role that past experiences play in decisions to use healthcare (see Galiatsatos and Hale 2016).

19. Friedland et al. 2012.

20. Metzl 2014. Drawing on his model, developing a health professions workforce will require five important skills: 1) the ability to identify social and structural factors underlying health, 2) the true integration of structural language into clinical practice, 3) the recognition that health disparities are not a result of cultural, but structural factors, 4) the identification of structural interventions to improve patient and community health, and 5) an acceptance that even well-intentioned community health programs sometimes miss the mark.

21. Chen et al. 2021.

22. See Institute of Medicine 1997.

23. American Hospital Association 2021.

24. In 2005, a letter from Grassley's office requested information from the IRS about "charitable activities, patient billing, and ventures with for-profit companies and hospitals" (Grassley 2015). In 2019, Sen. Grassley's office sent a letter to the IRS commissioner asking "for data on how many hospitals are in compliance with the requirements for tax exempt status and the status of IRS examinations of those not in compliance" (Grassley 2019). Among other things, Grassley pushed the IRS to show how it enforces the community benefit requirements for hospitals' non-profit status.

25. See Sanborn 2017.

26. American Hospital Association, n.d.

27. Berg 2010.

28. Ollove 2020.

29. See Ollove 2020; Wyland 2017.

30. An example of this occurred at the Cleveland Clinic. In the Clinic's 2016 Community Health Needs Assessment, the community listed infant mortality and its connection with long-standing structural racism as a top health need and yet the Clinic did not include any new programs to address this need in their community health planning for the next three years. Instead, the Clinic noted that it "cannot focus on or otherwise address the need for community services unrelated to the delivery of health care" (Cleveland Clinic 2016).

31. Franz, Skinner, and Murphy 2018.

32. Franz, Skinner, and Murphy 2018.

33. Tozzi 2021.

34. U.S. General Accountability Office 2020.

35. Atkeson and Higgins 2021.

36. Pennsylvania Department of State 1997.

37. Diamond 2017b.

38. Silverberg 2016; Bosch et al. 2018; Hannigan 1998.

39. Meisel and Pines 2008.

40. There is an extensive literature on the sociology of emergency department waiting rooms (see Burström et al. 2013).

41. Kenyon, Langley, and Paquin 2012.

42. Government Accounting Standards Board 2021.

43. Schiller 2018.

44. Chaskin and Joseph 2015.

45. Biron 2019.

46. International Association for Healthcare Security & Safety 2020.

47. Klinenberg 2018.

48. Kingdon 2011.

Appendix A

1. Du Bois 1898: 18, Itzigshon and Brown 2020.

2. Stainback, Tomaskovic-Devey, and Skaggs 2010.

3. Rothkopf 2009.

4. Deener 2020: 259.

5. Stinchcombe (1968) expressed concern over sociology's "generalizing impulse."

6. Brown-Saracino 2018: 254.

7. Glaser and Strauss 1967.

8. Reich 2016: 259.

9. Parker et al. 2019.

10. Duneier 1999.

11. Wynn 2015.

References

Acosta, Katie L. 2020. "Racism: A Public Health Crisis." *City & Community* 19(3):506–15.

Adams, Katie. 2021. "94% of Hospitals Still Noncompliant with Price Transparency Rule, Study Finds." *Becker's HealthCare*. https://www.beckershospitalreview.com/finance/94-of-hospitals -still-noncompliant-with-price-transparency-rule-study-finds.html. Accessed March 27, 2022.

Agency for Healthcare Research and Quality. 2017. "National Healthcare Quality and Disparities Report." https://www.ahrq.gov/sites/default/files/wysiwyg/research/findings/nhqrdr/2017 nhqdr.pdf. Accessed March 22, 2022.

Ahmed, Syed M., Joseph E. Kerschner, Mia C. DeFino, and Sharon N. Young. 2019. "Measuring Institutional Community Engagement: Adding Value to Academic Health Systems." *Journal of Clinical and Translational Science* 3(1):12–17.

Alexander, Brian. 2021. *The Hospital: Life, Death, and Dollars in a Small American Town.* New York: St. Martin's Press.

Allard, Scott W., and Mario L. Small. 2013. "Reconsidering the Urban Disadvantaged: The Role of Systems, Institutions, and Organizations." *ANNALS of the American Academy of Political and Social Science* 647(1):6–20.

Allen, Marian P., Robert E. Johnson, Evelyn Z. McClave, and Wilma Alvarado-Little. 2020. "Language, Interpretation, and Translation: A Clarification and Reference Checklist in Service of Health Literacy and Cultural Respect." *National Academy of Medicine.* https://nam.edu /language-interpretation-and-translation-a-clarification-and-reference-checklist-in-ser vice-of-health-literacy-and-cultural-respect/. Accessed March 22, 2022.

American Academy of Family Physicians. 2022. "AAFP Advocacy Focus: Graduate Medical Education (GME)." https://www.aafp.org/advocacy/advocacy-topics/physician-workforce/gme .html. Accessed March 28, 2022.

American Hospital Association. 2019. "Tax-Exempt Hospitals Provided $95 Billion in Total Benefits to Their Communities, Far Exceeding of the Value of Their Federal Tax Exemption: New Analysis." https://www.aha.org/press-releases/2019-05-22-new-analysis-tax-exempt -hospitals-provided-95-billion-total-benefits. Accessed December 22, 2022.

———. 2020. "COVID-19: Acknowledging and Addressing Racism and Xenophobia." https:// www.aha.org/resources/2020-06-03-covid-19-acknowledging-and-addressing-racism-and -xenophobia. Accessed December 22, 2022.

———. 2021. "Protecting Your Hospital's Tax-Exempt Status: Compliance with the Affordable Care Act and Final IRS Section 501(r) Regulations." https://www.aha.org/guidesreports/2018 -05-30-protecting-your-hospitals-tax-exempt-status. Accessed December 27, 2022.

———. 2022. "Fast Facts on U.S. Hospitals, 2022." https://www.aha.org/statistics/fast-facts-us -hospitals. Accessed March 21, 2022.

Andersen, Ronald M. 1995. "Revisiting the Behavioral Model and Access to Medical Care: Does It Matter?" *Journal of Health and Social Behavior* 36(1):1–10.

Anderson, Elijah. 2011. *The Cosmopolitan Canopy: Race and Civility in Everyday Life.* New York: W. W. Norton and Co.

Andrulis, Dennis P. 2006. "Access to High-Quality Health Care in U.S. Cities: Balancing Community Need and Service System Survival." In Nicholas Freudenberg, Sandro Galea, and David Vlahov, eds., *Cities and the Health of the Public.* Nashville: Vanderbilt University Press.

Andrzejewski, Thomas S., and David T. Abbott. 1977. "Clinic and UCI Accused of Land Squeeze." *The Plain Dealer* (A1), July 13.

Armstrong, David. 2020a. "Cleveland Hospitals' Private Police 'Border Patrol' Comes Under Scrutiny." *ProPublica.* https://www.propublica.org/article/cleveland-hospitals-private-police -border-patrol-comes-under-scrutiny. Accessed November 19, 2021.

———. 2020b. "The Startling Reach and Disparate Impact of Cleveland Clinic's Private Police Force." *ProPublica.* https://www.propublica.org/article/what-trump-and-biden-should-de bate-at-the-cleveland-clinic-why-the-hospitals-private-police-mostly-arrest-black-people. Accessed November 19, 2021.

Armstrong, Katrina, Abigail Rose, Nikki Peters, Judith A. Long, Suzanne McMurphy, and Judy A. Shea. 2006. "Distrust of the Health Care System and Self-Reported Health in the United States." *Journal of General Internal Medicine* 21(4):292–97.

Arnett, M. J., R. J. Thorpe, D. J. Gaskin, J. V. Bowie, and T. A. LaVeist. 2016. "Race, Medical Mistrust, and Segregation in Primary Care as Usual Source of Care: Findings from the Exploring Health Disparities in Integrated Communities Study." *Journal of Urban Health* 93(3):456–67.

Artiga, Samantha, and Elizabeth Hinton. 2018. *Beyond Health Care: The Role of Social Determinants in Promoting Health and Health Equity.* Kaiser Family Foundation. https://www.kff .org/disparities-policy/issue-brief/beyond-health-care-the-role-of-social-determinants-in -promoting-health-and-health-equity/. Accessed March 22, 2022.

Association of American Medical Colleges. 2020. "The Complexities of Physician Supply and Demand: Projections From 2018 to 2033." https://www.aamc.org/media/45976/download ?attachment. Accessed March 22, 2022.

Atkeson, Allie, and Elinor Higgins. 2021. "How States Can Hold Hospitals Accountable for Their Community Benefit Expenditures." *National Academy for State Health Policy* https://www .nashp.org/states-can-hold-hospitals-accountable-for-their-community-benefit-expendi tures/. Accessed March 22, 2022.

Auyero, Javier, and María Fernanda Berti. 2015. *In Harm's Way: The Dynamics of Urban Violence.* Princeton, NJ: Princeton University Press.

Bailey, Zinzi D., Nancy Krieger, Madina Agénor, Jasmine Graves, Natalia Linos, and Mary T. Bassett. 2017. "Structural Racism and Health Inequities in the USA: Evidence and Interventions." *The Lancet* 39(10077):1453–63.

Baker, Eileen F., Arthur R. Derse, Joel M. Geiderman, Kenneth V. Iserson, Catherine A. Marco, John C. Moskop, and ACEP Ethics Committee. 2016. "Law Enforcement and Emergency Medicine: An Ethical Analysis." *Annals of Emergency Medicine* 68(5):599–607.

Baldwin, Davarian L. 2021. *In the Shadow of the Ivory Tower: How Universities Are Plundering Our Cities.* New York: Bold Type Books.

Baltimore City Health Department. 2017. *Baltimore City Neighborhood Health Profile,* June. https://health.baltimorecity.gov/neighborhoods/neighborhood-health-profile-reports. Accessed March 22, 2022.

Barajas, Julia. 2020. "At Some U.S. Universities, A Time to Rethink Cops on Campus." *Los Angeles Times.* https://www.latimes.com/world-nation/story/2020-07-09/amid-nationwide-calls-to-de fund-the-police-universities-rethink-ties-to-police-dept. Accessed December 22, 2022.

Bartik, Timothy J., and George Erickcek. 2008. *The Local Economic Impact of "Eds & Meds": How Policies to Expand Universities and Hospitals Affect Metropolitan Economies.* Washington, DC: Brookings Institution.

Begun, James W., Linda M. Kahn, Brooke A. Cunningham, Jan K. Malcolm, and Sandra Potthoff. 2018. "A Measure of the Potential Impact of Hospital Community Health Activities on Population Health and Equity." *Journal of Public Health Management and Practice* 24(5):417–23.

Benit-Gbaffou, Claire, and Obvious Katsaura. 2014. "Community Leadership and the Construction of Political Legitimacy: Unpacking Bourdieu's 'Political Capital' in Post-Apartheid Johannesburg." *International Journal of Urban and Regional Research* 38(5):1807–32.

Bentley, Tanya G. K., Rachel M. Effros, Kartika Palar, and Emmett B. Keeler. 2008. "Waste in the U.S. Health Care System: A Conceptual Framework." *Milbank Quarterly* 86(4):629–59.

Berg, Jessica. 2010. "Putting the Community Back into the Community Benefit Standard." *Georgia Law Review* 44:375–431.

Berk, Marc L., and Claudia L. Schur. 2001. "The Effect of Fear on Access to Care among Undocumented Latino Immigrants." *Journal of Immigrant Health* 3(3):151–56.

Biron, Carey L. 2019. "'Good Neighbors'? U.S. Hospitals Invest in Land, Housing to Treat Crisis." *Reuters.* https://www.reuters.com/article/us-usa-housing-healthcare/good-neighbors-us-hos pitals-invest-in-land-housing-to-treat-crisis-idUSKBN1XV125. Accessed December 8, 2021.

Blair, Gifford, Larry Manheim, and Diane Cowper. 2002. "Unforeseen Policy Effects on the Safety Net: Medicaid, Private Hospital Closures and the Use of Local VAMCs." In *Social Inequalities, Health and Health Care Delivery* (Research in the Sociology of Health Care, Vol. 20), ed. Jennie Jacobs Kronenfeld, 45–55. Greenwich, CT: Emerald Group Publishing Limited.

Bohlen, Taegue. 2016. "Eight Things That Make Residents of Aurora Very, Very Mad." *Westword .com.* https://www.westword.com/arts/eight-things-that-make-residents-of-aurora-very-very -mad-7815361. Accessed September 4, 2021.

Bolon, Douglas S. 2005. "Comparing Mission Statement Content in For-Profit and Not-For-Profit Hospitals: Does Mission Really Matter?" *Hospital Topics* 83(4):2–9.

Bosch, Sheila J., Jason Meneely, Margaret Portillo, Candy Carmel-Gilfilen, Nam-Kyu Park, Maria Sanchez, Elizabeth Calienes, Robert Norberg, Abhinav Alakshendra, Jesse Anderson, Brandon Barnett, and Jessica VandeBiezen. 2018. "Mixed-Use Learning Zones for Millennials: A Typology for Bridging Learning from the Academe to the Profession." https://cdn .ymaws.com/www.edra.org/resource/resmgr/webpages/core/2018/Mixed-use_Learning .pdf. Accessed March 22, 2022.

Boulder Strong Resource Center. 2021. "How Our Neighbors in Aurora Are Helping Boulder Heal." May 26. https://wearebouldertrong.com/aurora-helping-boulder-heal/. Accessed December 13, 2021.

Boyd, Katherine. 2016. "The Origins of Hough." *Ideastream Public Media.* https://www.idea stream.org/news/the-origins-of-hough. Accessed March 22, 2022.

Brayne, Sarah. 2014. "Surveillance and System Avoidance: Criminal Justice Contact and Institutional Attachment." *American Sociological Review* 79(3):367–91.

Briggs, Laura. 2002. *Reproducing Empire: Race, Sex, Science, and U.S. Imperialism in Puerto Rico*. Berkeley: University of California Press.

Brown-Saracino, Japonica. 2009. *A Neighborhood That Never Changes: Gentrification, Social Preservation and the Search for Authenticity*. Chicago: University of Chicago Press.

———. 2018. *How Places Make Us*. Chicago: University of Chicago Press.

Bryson, Donna. 2019. "Aurora Approves More Money to Prevent Homelessness after a Motel Crisis Sparks a Successful Housing Program." *Denverite*. https://denverite.com/2019/12/10/after-a-crisis-at-a-motel-put-a-spotlight-on-housing-instability-in-aurora-the-denver-suburb-started-a-program-that-in-2-and-1-2-years-has-prevented-or-ended-homelessness-for-more-than-1000-houshold/. Accessed March 22, 2022.

Buchbinder, Mara. 2017. "Keeping Out and Getting In: Reframing Emergency Department Gatekeeping as Structural Competence." *Sociology of Health & Illness* 39(7):1166–79.

Buchheit, Bradley M., Erika L. Crable, Mari-Lynn Drainon, Sarah K. Lipson, and Alexander Y. Walley. 2021. "'Opening the Door to Somebody Who Has a Chance.'—The Experiences and Perceptions of Public Safety Personnel Towards a Public Restroom Overdose Prevention Alarm System." *International Journal of Drug Policy* 88:e103038.

Burke, Guenevere, and Julia Paradise. 2015. "Safety-Net Emergency Departments: A Look at Current Experiences and Challenges." *KFF*. https://www.kff.org/medicaid/issue-brief/safety-net-emergency-departments-a-look-at-current-experiences-and-challenges/. Accessed March 22, 2022.

Burström, Lena, Bengt Starrin, Marie-Louise Engström, and Hans Thulesius. 2013. "Waiting Management at the Emergency Department—A Grounded Theory Study." *BMC Health Services Research* 13(95).

Calhoun, Patricia. 2012. "Aurora Is Finally a Household Name . . . for the Wrong Reason." https://www.westword.com/news/aurora-is-finally-a-household-namefor-the-wrong-reason-5822506. Accessed March 22, 2022.

Call and Post. 1982. "Fire Inspections as a Weapon." *Call and Post* (Editorial), p. 8.

Campbell, Susan. 2019. *Frog Hollow: Stories from an American Neighborhood*. Middletown, CT: Wesleyan University Press.

Canada, Tracie, and Chelsey R. Carter. 2021. "The NFL's Racist 'Race Norming' Is an Afterlife of Slavery." *Scientific American*, July 8. https://www.scientificamerican.com/article/the-nfls-racist-race-norming-is-an-afterlife-of-slavery/.

Case Western Reserve University. n.d. "Fannie Lewis." *Encyclopedia of Cleveland History*. https://case.edu/ech/articles/l/lewis-fannie. Accessed March 22, 2022.

Catholic Health Association of the United States. 2009. "The IRS Form 990, Schedule H: Community Benefit and Catholic Health Care Governance Leaders." https://www.chausa.org/docs/default-source/general-files/form990_booklet-pdf.pdf. Accessed December 13, 2021.

Centers for Disease Control and Prevention. 2020. "QuickStats: Percentage of Deaths, by Place of Death—National Vital Statistics System, United States, 2000–2018." Morbidity and Mortality Weekly Report 69(19):611.

Centers for Medicare and Medicaid Services. 2021. "Emergency Medical Treatment & Labor Act (EMTALA)." https://www.cms.gov/Regulations-and-Guidance/Legislation/EMTALA. Accessed March 22, 2022.

———. n.d. "CMS' Value-Based Programs." https://www.cms.gov/medicare/quality-initiatives -patient-assessment-instruments/value-based-programs/value-based-programs.html. Accessed March 22, 2022.

———. n.d. "The Hospital Value-Based Purchasing (VBP) Program." https://www.cms.gov /Medicare/Quality-Initiatives-Patient-Assessment-Instruments/Value-Based-Programs /HVBP/Hospital-Value-Based-Purchasing. Accessed January 27, 2022.

———. n.d. "Translation and Interpretation Services." https://www.medicaid.gov/medicaid /financial-management/medicaid-administrative-claiming/translation-and-interpretation -services/index.html. Accessed January 27, 2022.

Chae, Duckhee H., Yun-Hee Park, Kyeong-Hwa Kang, and Tae-Hwa Lee. 2012. "A Study on Factors Affecting Cultural Competency of General Hospital Nurses." *Journal of Korean Academy of Nursing Administration* 18:76–86.

Chaskin, Robert J., and Mark L. Joseph. 2015. *Integrating the Inner City: The Promise and Perils of Mixed-Income Public Housing Transformation*. Chicago: University of Chicago Press.

Chen, Alice Hm, Mara K. Youdelman, and Jamie Brooks. 2007. "The Legal Framework for Language Access in Healthcare Settings: Title VI and Beyond." *Journal of General Internal Medicine* 22(Suppl 2):362–67.

Chen, Candice, Nicholas Chong, Quin Luo, and Jeongyoung Park. 2021. "Community Health Center Residency Training: Improving Staffing, Service, and Quality." *Family Medicine*. 53(8):689–96.

Chowkwanyun, Merlin. 2018. "Cleveland versus the Clinic: The 1960s Riots and Community Health Reform." *American Journal of Public Health* 108(11):1494–502.

Clarke, Amanda, Denis Martin, Derek Jones, Patricia Schofield, Geraldine Anthony, Paul McNamee, Denise Gray, and Blair H. Smith. 2014. "'I Try and Smile, I Try and Be Cheery, I Try Not to Be Pushy. I Try to Say "I'm Here for Help" but I Leave Feeling . . . Worried': A Qualitative Study of Perceptions of Interactions with Health Professionals by Community-Based Older Adults with Chronic Pain." *PLoS One* 9.9:e105450.

Cleveland Clinic. 2016. "Cleveland Clinic Main Campus 2016 CHNA and Implementation Strategy Report." https://my.clevelandclinic.org/about/community/reports/-/scassets/5ee8474c1 6e0423c8a8b098073f1bc99.ashx. Accessed January 15, 2022.

———. 2019. "Cleveland Clinic Main Campus CHNA and Implementation Strategy." https:// my.clevelandclinic.org/-/scassets/files/org/about/community-reports/chna/2019/2019-cleve land-clinic-main-campus-chna.pdf. Accessed October 16, 2022.

———. 2020a. "State of the Clinic." https://my.clevelandclinic.org/-/scassets/files/org/about/who -we-are/state-of-the-clinic.pdf. Accessed December 13, 2021.

———. 2020b. "School of Diagnostic Imaging Cleveland Clinic Health System: The Jeanne Clery Act, Annual Safety and Security Report 2020." http://portals.clevelandclinic.org/Portals/98 /SDIAnnualSecurityReport2020.pdf. Accessed March 22, 2022.

———. 2021. "Creating an Environment That Embraces Diversity, Inclusion and Equity: Programs and Partnerships Focus on Community, Diverse Hiring." https://consultqd.cleve landclinic.org/creating-an-environment-that-embraces-diversity-inclusion-and-equity/. Accessed December 13, 2021.

———. n.d. "Police & Security." https://my.clevelandclinic.org/patients/visitor-information /police-security. Accessed February 19, 2022.

Cleveland Department of Health. n.d. "Infant Mortality within Cleveland: An In-Depth Analysis (2012–2015)." https://www.clevelandhealth.org/assets/documents/health/health_statistics /2012-2015_Infant_Mortality_Report.pdf. Accessed December 21, 2022.

Cleveland Foundation. 2014. *Building a 21st Century City through the Power of Anchor Insti-tution Collaboration.* https://policycommons.net/artifacts/1643557/building-a-21st-century-city-through-the-power-of-anchor-institution-collaboration/. Accessed March 22, 2022.

Cleveland Restoration Society. n.d. "Know Your Heritage—The Great Migration." https://www.clevelandrestoration.org/projects/the-african-american-experience-in-cleveland/the-great-migration. Accessed February 3, 2022.

Clifton, Brad. n.d. "The Cleveland Clinic X-Ray Fire of 1929." *Cleveland Historical* https://cleve landhistorical.org/items/show/573. Accessed February 3, 2022.

Clouette, Bruce, and Brian Lever. 2004. *The Healing Triangle: Hartford Hospital's First 150 Years.* Hartford, CT: Hartford Hospital.

Clough, John D. 2004. *To Act as a Unit: The Cleveland Clinic Story.* 4th ed. Cleveland: Cleveland Clinic Press.

Collins, Randall. 2004. *Interaction Ritual Chains.* Princeton, NJ: Princeton University Press.

Committee on Accounting for Socioeconomic Status in Medicare Payment Programs. 2016. *Accounting for Social Risk Factors in Medicare Payment: Data.* Washington, DC: National Academies Press. https://www.ncbi.nlm.nih.gov/books/NBK395663/. Accessed December 22, 2022.

Commonwealth Fund. 2020. "U.S. Health Insurance Coverage in 2019: A Looming Crisis In Affordability." https://www.commonwealthfund.org/publications/issue-briefs/2020/aug/looming-crisis-health-coverage-2020-biennial#:~:text=In%20the%20first%20half%20of%202020%2C%2043.4%20percent%20of%20U.S.,uninsured%20rate%20was%2012.5%20percent. Accessed September 4, 2021.

Comfort, Megan. 2007. "Punishment beyond the Legal Offender." *Annual Review of Law and Social Science* 3:271–96.

Connecticut General Assembly. 2019. *Testimony of Pamela Clark, R.N. Nurse Manager.* https://www.cga.ct.gov/2019/APPdata/Tmy/2019HB-07148-R000305-DSS-Hartford%20Healthcare-Brownstone%20-%20Clark%20-%20Pamela-TMY.pdf. Accessed February 20, 2022.

Corburn, James. 2005. *Street Science: Community Knowledge and Environmental Health Justice.* Cambridge, MA: MIT Press.

Cowan, Spencer M., William Rohe, and Esmail Baku. 1999. "Factors Influencing the Performance of Community Development Corporations." *Journal of Urban Affairs* 21:325–39.

Cowan, Tadlock, and Baird Webel. 2005. "Congressional Research Service. Military Base Closure: Socioeconomic Impacts." *Congressional Research Service* RS22147.

Cronin, Corey E., and Douglas S. Bolon. 2018. "Comparing Hospital Mission Statement Content in a Changing Healthcare Field." *Hospital Topics* 96(1):28–34.

Crosson, Francis J. 2011. "The Accountable Care Organization: Whatever Its Growing Pains, the Concept Is Too Vitally Important to Fail." *Health Affairs* 30(7):1250–55.

Cruz, Jose. 1998. *Identity and Power: Puerto Rican Politics and the Challenge of Ethnicity.* Philadelphia: Temple University Press.

Cuyahoga County Board of Health. 2021. "Preliminary 2020 Cuyahoga County Infant Mortality & Birth Outcome Data." https://www.firstyearcleveland.org/files/assets/yearend202010.6.21.pdf. Accessed March 22, 2022.

Davidson, Mark, and Kevin Ward. 2018. *Cities Under Austerity: Restructuring the US Metropolis.* Albany: State University of New York Press.

Dawn Clinic. 2022. "About DAWN." https://www.dawnhealth.org/about-dawn. Accessed December 22, 2022.

Day, Meagan. 2021. "The Rise of the UniverCity: An Interview with Davarian Baldwin." *Jacobin*. https://jacobinmag.com/2021/09/university-cities-urban-development-gentrification. Accessed December 13, 2021.

De Avila, Joseph. 2017. "Hartford's Finances Spotlight Property-Tax Quandary." *Wall Street Journal*. https://www.wsj.com/articles/hartfords-finances-spotlight-property-tax-quandary-1496750405. Accessed March 22, 2022.

DeBoer, Freddie. n.d. "Hartford, Connecticut." *N+1*. https://www.nplusonemag.com/online-only/city-by-city/hartford-connecticut. Accessed December 22, 2022.

Deener, Andrew. 2020. *The Problem with Feeding Cities*. Chicago: University of Chicago Press.

DeJesus, Jeannette B. 2009. "Health Care Interpreters: Medical Necessity." *Hartford Courant*. http://www.hartfordinfo.org/issues/documents/health/htfd_courant_031309.asp. Accessed March 22, 2022.

De Lisle, Kate, Teresa Litton, Allison Brennan, and David Muhlestein. 2017. "The 2017 ACO Survey: What Do Current Trends Tell Us About the Future of Accountable Care?" *Health Affairs Blog*. https://www.healthaffairs.org/do/10.1377/forefront.20171021.165999/full/. Accessed March 22, 2022.

Democracy Collaborative. n.d. "Hospitals Aligned for Health Communities: Toolkits to Help Hospitals and Health Systems Build Community Wealth through Inclusive Hiring, Investment, and Purchasing." https://hospitaltoolkits.org. Accessed February 18, 2022.

Desmond, Matthew. 2016. *Evicted: Poverty and Profit in the American City*. New York: Crown.

Detrow, Scott, and Elisabeth Rosenthal. 2021. "A Hospital Hiked the Price of a Routine Childbirth by Calling It an 'Emergency.'" *Shots: Health News from NPR*, October 27. https://www.npr.org/transcripts/1049138668?ft=nprml&f=488995557.

Diamond, Dan. 2017a. "How the Cleveland Clinic Grows Healthily While Its Neighbors Stay Sick." *Politico*. https://www.politico.com/interactives/2017/obamacare-cleveland-clinic-non-profit-hospital-taxes. Accessed September 4, 2021.

———. 2017b. "Cleveland Clinic CEO Toby Cosgrove on What He's Telling His Senator, and News Roundup." *PulseCheck*, June 29. https://politicos-pulse-check.simplecast.com/episodes/cleveland-clinic-ceo-toby-cosgrove-on. Accessed March 22, 2022.

Donnan, Shawn. 2020. "Cleveland Clinic Thrives While Its Black Neighbors Fall Behind." *Bloomberg Businessweek*. https://www.bloomberg.com/news/features/2020-09-29/cleveland-clinic-presidential-debate-sponsor-faces-tough-questions-on-race. Accessed March 22, 2022.

Drees, Laurie Meijer. 2013. *Healing Histories: Stories from Canada's Indian Hospitals*. Edmonton, Canada: University of Alberta Press.

Du Bois, W. E. B. 1898. "The Study of Negro Problems." *Annals of the American Academy of Political and Social Science* 11:1–23.

———. 1899. *The Philadelphia Negro: A Social Study*. Philadelphia: University of Pennsylvania Press.

———. 1946. *The World and Africa: An Inquiry into the Part Which Africa Has Played in World History*. New York: Viking Press.

Dubb, Steve, Sarah McKinley, and Ted Howard. 2013. *Achieving the Anchor Promise: Improving Outcomes for Low-Income Children, Families and Communities*. Annie E. Casey Foundation and Democracy Collaborative, at the University of Maryland.

Duneier, Mitchell. 1999. *Sidewalk*. New York: Farrar, Straus & Giroux.

Edgar, John. 2018. "Getting Ahead of Gentrification in the South Side of Columbus." *Shelterforce*, May 7. https://shelterforce.org/2018/05/07/building-a-sustainable-mixed-income-community-in-south-side-columbus. Accessed March 21, 2022.

Ergungor, O. Emre, and Nelson Oliver. 2013. "The Employability of Returning Citizens Is Key to Neighborhood Revitalization." *Federal Reserve Bank of Cleveland*, issue 11.

Erickson, David. 2013. "Linking Community Development and Health." Robert Wood Johnson Foundation. http://www.rwjf.org/content/dam/farm/reports/reports/2013/rwjf406408. Accessed August 25, 2021.

Erickson, David, and Nancy Andrews. 2011. "Partnerships among Community Development, Public Health, and Health Care Could Improve the Well-Being of Low-Income People." *Health Affairs* 30(11):2056–63.

Etienne, Harley. 2012. *Pushing Back the Gates: Neighborhood Perspectives on University-Driven Revitalization in West Philadelphia*. Philadelphia: Temple University Press.

Evans-Pritchard, Ambrose. 2011. "Spain's Astonishing Co-Op Takes on the World." *The Telegraph*. https://www.telegraph.co.uk/finance/economics/8329355/Spains-astonishing-co-op -takes-on-the-world.html. Accessed December 13, 2021.

Fairfax Renaissance. 2020. "Welcome to Fairfax Workforce Redevelopment Program." https:// fairfaxrenaissance.org/workforce-development/. Accessed September 4, 2021.

Farrer, James. 2011. "Global Nightscapes in Shanghai as Ethnosexual Contact Zones." *Journal of Ethnic and Migration Studies* 37(5):747–64.

Feagin, Joe, and Zinobia Bennefield. 2014. "Systemic Racism and U.S. Health Care." *Social Science & Medicine* 103:7–14.

Federal Reserve Bank of Cleveland. 2019. "Cleveland—Slow Growth and Falling Unemployment." August 5. https://www.clevelandfed.org/newsroom-and-events/press-releases/2019 /pr-20190805-cleveland-metro-mix. Accessed December 22, 2022.

Fentress, James, and Chris Wickham. 1992. *Social Memory*. Oxford: Blackwell Publishers.

Fink, Sheri. 2013. *Five Days at Memorial: Life and Death in a Storm-Ravaged Hospital*. New York: Crown.

Finkler, Kaja, Cynthia Hunter, and Rick Iedema. 2008. "What Is Going On? Ethnography in Hospital Spaces." *Journal of Contemporary Ethnography* 37(2):246–50.

Flores, Glenn. 2005. "The Impact of Medical Interpreter Services on the Quality of Health Care: A Systematic Review." *Medical Care Research and Review* 62(3):255–99.

Flores, Glenn, Milagros Abreu, Cara Pizzo Barone, Richard Bachur, and Hua Lin. 2012. "Errors of Medical Interpretation and Their Potential Clinical Consequences: A Comparison of Professional versus Ad Hoc versus No Interpreters." *Annals of Emergency Medicine* 60(5):545–53.

Foust, D., and K. J. Rhee. 1993. "The Incidence of Battery in an Urban Emergency Department." *Annals of Emergency Medicine* 22(3):583–85.

Frank, Richard G., and David S. Salkever. 1991. "The Supply of Charity Services by Nonprofit Hospitals: Motives and Market Structure." *The RAND Journal of Economics* 22(3):430–45.

Franz, Berkeley, Kelly Choyke, Cory E. Cronin, Janet E. Simon, Maxwell T. Hall, and Vanessa Rodriguez. 2021. "For-Profit Hospitals as Anchor Institutions in the United States: A Study of Organizational Stability." *BMC Health Services Research* 21:1326.

Franz, Berkeley, Ben Parker, Adrienne Milner, and Jomills H. Braddock II. 2021. "The Relationship between Systemic Racism, Residential Segregation, and Racial/Ethnic Disparities in COVID-19 Deaths in the United States." *Ethnicity & Disease* 32(1):31–38.

Franz, Berkeley A., Daniel Skinner, and John W. Murphy. 2018. "Defining 'Community' in Community Health Evaluation: Perspectives from a Sample of Nonprofit Appalachian Hospitals." *American Journal of Evaluation* 39(2):237–56.

Franz, Berkeley, Daniel Skinner, Jonathan Wynn, and Kelly Kelleher. 2019. "Urban Hospitals as Anchor Institutions: Frameworks for Medical Sociology." *Socius*, 5. Online first.

Freidson, Eliot. 1963. *The Hospital in Modern Society*. New York: The Free Press of Glencoe.

———. 1970. *Profession of Medicine: A Study of the Sociology of Applied Knowledge*. Chicago: University of Chicago Press.

Friedland, Allen, Hayley C. Rintel-Queller, Devi Unnikrishnan, and David A. Paul. 2012. "Field Trips as a Novel Means of Experiential Learning in Ambulatory Pediatrics." *Journal of Graduate Medical Education* 4(2):246–49.

Fukuyama, Francis 1995. *Trust: The Social Virtues and The Creation of Prosperity*. New York: The Free Press.

Galiatsatos, Panagis, and W. Daniel Hale. 2016. "Promoting Health and Wellness in Congregations Through Lay Health Educators: A Case Study of Two Churches." *Journal of Religion and Health* 55(1):288–95.

Gamble, Vanessa Northington. 1997. "Under the Shadow of Tuskegee: African Americans and Health Care." *American Journal of Public Health* 87(3):1773–78.

Garmon, Christopher, and Benjamin Chartock. 2017. "One in Five Inpatient Emergency Department Cases May Lead to Surprise Bills." *Health Affairs* 36(1):177–81.

Garran, Ann Marie, and Brian M. Rasmussen. 2019. "How Should Organizations Respond to Racism Against Health Care Workers?" *AMA Journal of Ethics* 21(6):E499–504.

Gaskin, Darrell J, Roland J. Thorpe Jr., Emma E. McGinty, Kelly Bower, Charles Rohde, J. Hunter Young, Thomas A. LaVeist, and Lisa Dubay. 2014. "Disparities in Diabetes: The Nexus of Race, Poverty, and Place." *American Journal of Public Health* 104(11):2147–55.

Geertz, Clifford. 1983. *Local Knowledge*. New York: Basic Books.

Georgetown University. 2016. "Georgetown Shares Slavery, Memory, and Reconciliation Report, Racial Justice Steps." https://www.georgetown.edu/slavery-memory-reconciliation-working -group-sept-2016. Accessed March 22, 2022.

Geronimus, Arline T., John Bound, Timothy Waidmann, Cynthia G. Colen, and Dianne Steffick. 2001. "Inequality in Life Expectancy, Functional Status, and Active Life Expectancy across Selected Black and White Populations in the United States." *Demography* 38:227–51.

Glaser, Barney G., and Anselm L. Strauss. 1967. *The Discovery of Grounded Theory: Strategies for Qualitative Research*. London: Aldine Publishing Company.

Glaser, Susan. 2016. "Cleveland's InterContinental Hotel Renovates Presidential Suite; Will Trump Stay Here?" https://www.cleveland.com/travel/2016/07/clevelands_intercontinental _ho.html. Accessed March 22, 2022.

Goffman, Alice. 2014. *On the Run: Fugitive Life in an American City*. Chicago: University of Chicago Press.

Goffman, Erving. 1974. *Frame Analysis: An Essay on the Organization of Experience*. Cambridge, MA: Harvard University Press.

Gold, Jenny. 2012. "New Rules Will Ban ER Debt Collections at Charitable Hospitals." *Kaiser Health News*. https://khn.org/news/er-debt-charity-hospitals/. Accessed December 13, 2021.

Gonzales, Teresa. 2021. *Building a Better Chicago: Race and Community Resistance to Urban Development*. New York: NYU Press.

Goodson, Leigh, and Matt Vassar. 2011. "An Overview of Ethnography in Healthcare and Medical Education Research." *Journal of Educational Evaluation for Health Professions* 8:4.

Gordon, James A. 1999. "The Hospital Emergency Department as a Social Welfare Institution." *Annals of Emergency Medicine* 33(3):321–25.

Gosselin, Kenneth R. 2017. "Hartford's Newest Residence, Capitol Lofts, Already Half Full." *Hartford Courant.* https://www.courant.com/business/hc-capitol-lofts-grand-opening-2017 0426-story.html. Accessed March 22, 2022.

Government Accounting Standards Board. 2021. "About the GASB." https://www.gasb.org/about gasb. September. Accessed December 8, 2021.

Graham, Garth, Mary Lynn Ostrowski, and Alyse Sabina. 2015. "Defeating the ZIP Code Health Paradigm: Data, Technology, And Collaboration Are Key." *Health Affairs Blog.*

Grassley, Charles. 2015. "Grassley Asks Non-Profit Hospitals to Account for Activities Related to Their Tax-Exempt Status." https://www.grassley.senate.gov/news/news-releases/grassley-asks -non-profit-hospitals-account-activities-related-their-tax-exempt. Accessed March 22, 2022.

———. 2019. "Grassley Renews Probe of Non-Profit, Tax-Exempt Hospitals." https://www.grass ley.senate.gov/news/news-releases/grassley-renews-probe-non-profit-tax-exempt-hospitals. Accessed March 22, 2022.

Green, Carmen R., Wayne R. McCullough, and Jamie D. Hawley. 2018. "Visiting Black Patients: Racial Disparities in Security Standby Requests." *Journal of the National Medical Association* 110(1):37–43.

Green, Chuck. 2015. "Hospitals Turn to Just-in-Time Buying to Control Supply Chain Costs." *Healthcare Finance.* https://www.healthcarefinancenews.com/news/hospitals-turn-just-time -buying-control-supply-chain-costs. Accessed March 22, 2022.

Greenberg, Miriam. 2000. "Branding Cities: A Social History of the Urban Lifestyle Magazine." *Urban Affairs Review* 36(2):228–63.

Greene, Jessica, Jan Blustein, and Beth C. Weitzman. 2006. "Race, Segregation, and Physicians' Participation in Medicaid." *Milbank Quarterly* 84(2):239–72.

Greenwood-Ericksen, Margaret B., and Keith Kocher. 2019. "Trends in Emergency Department Use by Rural and Urban Populations in the United States." *JAMA Network Open* 2(4):e191919.

Grzegorek, Vince. 2018. "Employee-Owned Evergreen Cooperative Laundry Takes Over Cleve-land Clinic Laundry Operation, Adding 100 Workers to Coop." *Cleveland Scene.* https:// www.clevescene.com/scene-and-heard/archives/2018/05/10/employee-owned-evergreen -cooperative-laundry-takes-over-cleveland-clinic-laundry-operation-adding-100-workers -to-coop. Accessed August 26, 2021.

Hagaman, Frank. 2016. "The (Reborn) Perfect Six." *Hartford Preservation Alliance.* https://www .hartfordpreservation.org/reborn-perfect-six. Accessed September 4, 2021.

Hakala, Ulla, Arja Lemmetyinen, and Jürgen Gnoth. 2010. *Case A: The Role of Nokia in Branding Finland—Companies as Vectors of Nation Branding.* New York: Palgrave Macmillan.

Hannigan, John. 1998. *Fantasy City: Pleasure and Profit in the Postmodern Metropolis.* London and New York: Routledge.

Harder, Ben. 2021. "America's Best Hospitals: The 2021–2022 Honor Roll." *U.S. News & World Report.* https://health.usnews.com/health-care/best-hospitals/articles/best-hospitals-honor -roll-and-overview. Accessed March 25, 2022.

Hartford HealthCare. 2018. "Hartford Region Update on Community Health Improvement Plan." June 25, 2018. https://hartfordhealthcare.org/file%20library/chna/chip-2018-hartford -region.pdf.

———. 2021. "Hartford Hospital, 2021: Community Health Needs Assessment." https://hartford healthcare.org/file%20library/chna/chna-hh-2021.pdf.

———. n.d. "Social Work." https://hartfordhospital.org/patients-and-visitors/for-patients/so cial-work-services. Accessed January 25, 2022.

Health Research & Educational Trust. 2017. "Social Determinants of Health Series: Transportation and the Role of Hospitals." *American Hospital Association* http://www.hpoe.org/Reports-HPOE/2017/sdoh-transportation-role-of-hospitals.pdf. Accessed March 22, 2022.

Health Resources and Services Administration. n.d. "What Is Shortage Designation?" https://bhw.hrsa.gov/shortage-designation/muap. Accessed March 2, 2022.

Helmuth, Laura. 2013. "Why Are You Not Dead Yet?" *Slate.com.* https://slate.com/technology/2013/09/life-expectancy-history-public-health-and-medical-advances-that-lead-to-long-lives.html. Accessed September 4, 2021.

Henderson, Heather, Stephanie Child, Spencer Moore, Justin B. Moore, and Andrew T. Kaczynski. 2016. "The Influence of Neighborhood Aesthetics, Safety, and Social Cohesion on Perceived Stress in Disadvantaged Communities." *American Journal of Community Psychology* 58:80–88.

Henderson, Thomas M. 2021. "How Accountable to the Public Is Funding for Graduate Medical Education? The Case for State Medicaid GME Payments." *American Journal of Public Health* 111(7):1216–19.

Hernandez, Sarah Gabriella, Ana Genkova, Yvette Castañeda, Simone Alexander, and Jennifer Hebert-Beirne. 2017. "Oral Histories as Critical Qualitative Inquiry in Community Health Assessment." *Health Education & Behavior* 44(5):705–15.

Hexter, Kathryn W., Candi Clouse, Nick Downer, and Liam Robinson. 2017. "Greater University Circle Initiative: Year 6 Evaluation Report." *Urban Publications.* https://engagedscholarship.csuohio.edu/urban_facpub/1497. Accessed March 27, 2022.

Himmelstein, David U., and Steffie Woolhandler. 2016. "Public Health's Falling Share of US Health Spending." *American Journal of Public Health* 106(1):56–57.

Hirschman, Daniel, and Isaac Ariail Reed. 2014. "Formation Stories and Causality in Sociology." *Sociological Theory* 32(4):259–82.

Hogg, Rachel A., Glen P. Mays, and Cezar B. Mamaril. 2015. "Hospital Contributions to the Delivery of Public Health Activities in US Metropolitan Areas: National and Longitudinal Trends." *American Journal of Public Health* 105(8):1646–52.

Hooker, Kenneth. 1974. "Mother Files Suit Against 2 Hospitals." *Hartford Courant,* p. 3.

Hughes, C. J. 2016. "Trading Hospital Rooms for Hotel Suites." *New York Times,* December 20.

Hughes, Michelle M., et al. 2021. "County-Level COVID-19 Vaccination Coverage and Social Vulnerability—United States, December 14, 2020–March 1, 2021." *Morbidity and Mortality Weekly Report* 70:431–36.

Hunt, Bijou R., Gary Tran, and Steven Whitman. 2015. "Life Expectancy Varies in Local Communities in Chicago: Racial and Spatial Disparities and Correlates." *Journal of Racial and Ethnic Health Disparities* 2:425–33.

Hunter, Marcus Anthony, and Zandria Robinson. 2018. *Chocolate Cities: The Black Map of American Life.* Berkeley: University of California Press.

Hussein, Mustafa, Ana V. Diez Roux, and Robert I. Field. 2016. "Neighborhood Socioeconomic Status and Primary Health Care: Usual Points of Access and Temporal Trends in a Major US Urban Area." *Journal of Urban Health: Bulletin of the New York Academy of Medicine* 93(6):1027–45.

Hyra, Derek. 2012. "Conceptualizing the New Urban Renewal: Comparing the Past to the Present." *Urban Affairs Review* 48(4):498–527.

Illescas, Carlos. 2016. "Aurora Struggles to Find an Identity beyond the Grit of East Colfax." *Denver Post.* Accessed March 22, 2022.

Initiative for a Competitive Inner City. 2016. "What Works for Cities: Will Hospitals Become the New Vanguard in Urban Economic Development?" http://icic.org/wp-content/uploads/2016 /04/ICIC_WW_Hospital_Anchors_Final_Updated.pdf. Accessed December 22, 2022.

Institute of Medicine. 1997. "Appendix B, History and Current Status of Medicare Graduate Medical Education Funding." https://www.ncbi.nlm.nih.gov/books/NBK233563/. Accessed March 22, 2022.

Institute of Medicine Committee on Understanding and Eliminating Racial and Ethnic Dispari- ties in Health Care. 2003. *Unequal Treatment: Confronting Racial and Ethnic Disparities in Health Care*, ed. Brian D. Smedley, Adrienne Y. Stith, and Alan R. Nelson. Washington, DC: National Academies Press.

Internal Revenue Service. 1969. Revenue Ruling 69–545. https://www.irs.gov/pub/irs-tege/rr69 -545.pdf.

———. 2014. "Instructions for Schedule H (Form 990)." Washington, DC: IRS; December 22. Cited April 27, 2015. https://www.irs.gov/pub/irs-pdf/i990sh.pdf.

———. n.d. "Charitable Hospitals—General Requirements for Tax-Exemption Under Sect- ion 501(c)(3)." https://www.irs.gov/charities-non-profits/charitable-hospitals-general-require ments-for-tax-exemption-under-section-501c3. Accessed January 21, 2022.

———. n.d. "Requirements for 501(c)(3) Hospitals Under the Affordable Care Act—Section 501(r)." https://www.irs.gov/charities-non-profits/charitable-organizations/requirements-for-501c3 -hospitals-under-the-affordable-care-act-section-501r. Accessed March 24, 2022.

International Association for Healthcare Security & Safety. 2020. "IAHSS Foundation's 2020 Healthcare Crime Survey." https://iahssf.org/assets/2020-Healthcare-Crime-Survey-IAHSS -Foundation.pdf. Accessed December 8, 2021.

Itzigsohn, José, and Karida L. Brown. 2020. *The Sociology of W. E. B. Du Bois: Racialized Moder- nity and the Global Color Line*. New York: NYU Press.

Jacoby, Sara F., Therese S. Richmond, Daniel N. Holena, and Elinore J. Kaufman. 2018. "A Safe Haven for the Injured? Urban Trauma Care at the Intersection of Healthcare, Law Enforce- ment, and Race." *Social Science & Medicine* 199:115–22.

John, Mark. 2021. "Public Trust Crumbles under COVID-19, Fake News: Survey." *Reuters,* Jan- uary 13. https://www.reuters.com/article/us-health-coronavirus-global-trust/public-trust -crumbles-under-covid-19-fake-news-survey-idUSKBN29I0NL. Accessed March 22, 2022.

Johns Hopkins Hub. 2020. "Johns Hopkins Will Pause Development of a Police Department for at Least Two Years." https://hub.jhu.edu/2020/06/12/hopkins-pauses-jhpd-for-at-least-two -years/. Accessed December 23, 2022.

Johns Hopkins Medicine. n.d. "Honoring Henrietta Lacks." https://www.hopkinsmedicine.org /henriettalacks/honoring-henrietta-lacks.html. Accessed December 22, 2022.

Johnson, Pamela Jo, Neha Ghildayal, Andrew C. Ward, Bjorn C. Westgard, Lori L. Boland, and Jon S. Hokanson. 2012. "Disparities in Potentially Avoidable Emergency Department (ED) Care: ED Visits for Ambulatory Care Sensitive Conditions." *Medical Care* 50(12):1020–28.

Jones, Kristin. 2015. "Undocumented Immigrants Struggle to Find Care." *Post Independent,* April 20. https://www.postindependent.com/news/local/undocumented-immigrants-struggle-to -find-care/. Accessed March 22, 2022.

Juckett, Gregory, and Kendra Unger. 2014. "Appropriate Use of Medical Interpreters." *American Family Physician* 90(7):476–80.

Kaiser Family Foundation. 2021. "Surprise Medical Bills: New Protections for Consumers Take Effect in 2022." February 4. https://www.kff.org/private-insurance/fact-sheet/surprise

-medical-bills-new-protections-for-consumers-take-effect-in-2022/. Accessed December 12, 2021.

Kao, Audiey. 2001. "Disparity in Health: Is Geography Destiny?" *AMA Journal of Ethics*. https://journalofethics.ama-assn.org/article/disparity-health-geography-destiny/2001-06. Accessed December 21, 2022.

Kenyon, Daphne A., Adam H. Langley, and Bethany P. Paquin. 2012. "Rethinking Property Tax Incentives for Business." *Lincoln Institute on Land Policy*. https://www.lincolninst.edu/sites/default/files/pubfiles/rethinking-property-tax-incentives-for-business-full_0.pdf. Accessed January 6, 2022.

Kershaw, Kiarri N., Whitney R. Robinson, Penny Gordon-Larsen, Margaret T. Hicken, David C. Goff Jr., Mercedes R. Carnethon, Catarina I. Kiefe, Stephen Sidney, and Ana V. Diez Roux. 2017. "Association of Changes in Neighborhood-Level Racial Residential Segregation with Changes in Blood Pressure Among Black Adults: The CARDIA Study." *JAMA Internal Medicine* 177(7):996–1002.

King, Robert. 2020. "Mayo Clinic CEO Blasts 'Just-in-Time' Ordering as Pandemic Changes Supply Chain." July 7. https://www.fiercehealthcare.com/hospitals/mayo-clinic-ceo-blasts-just-time-ordering-as-pandemic-changes-supply-chain. Accessed March 22, 2022.

Kingdon, John. 2011. *Agendas, Alternatives, and Public Policies*, 2nd ed. Boston: Longman.

Kirby, Russell S. 2017. "The US Black-White Infant Mortality Gap: Marker of Deep Inequities." *American Journal of Public Health* 107(5):644–45.

Kisacky, Jeanne. 2017. *Rise of the Modern Hospital: An Architectural History of Health and Healing*. Pittsburgh: University of Pittsburgh Press.

Kleinman, Arthur. 2015. "Care: In Search of a Health Agenda." *The Lancet* 386(9990):240–41.

Klinenberg, Eric. 2018. *Palaces for the People: How Social Infrastructure Can Help Fight Inequality, Polarization, and the Decline of Civic Life*. New York: Penguin.

Kocher, Bob, and Rahul Rajkumar. 2021. "Setting the Stage for the Next 10 Years of Health Care Payment Innovation." *Journal of the American Medical Association* 326(10):905–6.

Koh, Howard K., Amy Bantham, Alan C. Geller, Mark A. Rukavina, Karen M. Emmons, Pamela Yatsko, and Robert Restuccia. 2020. "Anchor Institutions: Best Practices to Address Social Needs and Social Determinants of Health." *American Journal of Public Health* 110:309–16.

Komarnisky, Sara, Paul Hackett, Sylvia Abonyi, Courtney Heffernan, and Richard Long. 2016. "'Years Ago': Reconciliation and First Nations Narratives of Tuberculosis in the Canadian Prairie Provinces." *Critical Public Health* 26(4):381–93.

Kotecki, Jack A., Keith P. Gennuso, Marjory L. Givens, and David A. Kindig. 2019. "Separate and Sick: Residential Segregation and the Health of Children and Youth in Metropolitan Statistical Areas." *Journal of Urban Health* 96:149–58.

Krieger, James, David E. Jacobs, Peter J. Ashley, Andrea Baeder, Ginger L. Chew, Dorr Dearborn, H. Patricia Hynes, J. David Miller, Rebecca Morlley, Felicia Rabito, Darryl C. Zeldin, et al. 2010. "Housing Interventions and Control of Asthma-Related Indoor Biologic Agents: A Review of the Evidence." *Journal of Public Health Management and Practice* 16 (5 Suppl.): S11–20.

Lao-Montes, Agustin. 2007. "Decolonial Moves: Trans-Locating African Diasporic Spaces." *Cultural Studies* 21(2):309–38.

Lara-Millán, Armando. 2014. "Public Emergency Room Overcrowding in the Era of Mass Imprisonment." *American Sociological Review* 79(5):866–87.

———. 2021. *Redistributing the Poor: Jails, Hospitals, and the Crisis of Law and Fiscal Austerity*. Oxford: Oxford University Press.

Largent, Emily A. 2018. "Public Health, Racism, and the Lasting Impact of Hospital Segregation." *Public Health Reports* 133(6):715–20.

Laurencin, Cato T. 2021. "Addressing Justified Vaccine Hesitancy in the Black Community." *Journal of Racial and Ethnic Health Disparities* 8:543–46.

LaVeist, Thomas A., Lydia A. Isaac, and Karen Patricia Williams. 2009. "Mistrust of Health Care Organizations Is Associated with Underutilization of Health Services." *Health Services Research* 44(6):2093–105.

LaVeist, Thomas A., Kim J. Nickerson, and Janice V. Bowie. 2000. "Attitudes about Racism, Medical Mistrust, and Satisfaction with Care among African American and White Cardiac Patients." *Medical Care Research and Review* 57(1_suppl):146–61.

Lazarus, Barry A. 1991. "The Practice of Medicine and Prejudice in a New England Town: The Founding of Mount Sinai Hospital, Hartford, Connecticut." *Journal of American Ethnic History* 10(3):21–41.

Leblang, David, and Satyanath Shanker. 2006. "Institutions, Expectations, and Currency Crises." *International Organization* 60(1):245–62.

Leitner, Helga. 2012. "Spaces of Encounters: Immigration, Race, Class, and the Politics of Belonging in Small-Town America." *Annals of the Association of American Geographers* 102:828–46.

Lie, Désirée A., Elizabeth Lee-Rey, Art Gomez, Sylvia Bereknyei, and Clarence H. Braddock. 2011. "Does Cultural Competency Training of Health Professionals Improve Patient Outcomes? A Systematic Review and Proposed Algorithm for Future Research." *Journal of General Internal Medicine* 26(3):317–25.

Liou, Y. Thomas, and Robert C. Stroh. 1998. "Community Development Intermediary Systems in the United States: Origins, Evolution, and Functions." *Housing Policy Debate* 9(3):575–94.

Lipsitz, George. 2011. *How Racism Takes Place*. Philadelphia: Temple University Press.

Litt, Steven. 2019. "Cleveland to Roll Out Opportunity Corridor Plans Showing How Neighborhoods Could Benefit." *Cleveland.com*. https://www.cleveland.com/architecture/2017/07/cleveland_to_roll_out_opportun.html. Accessed September 4, 2021.

Logan, John R., and Harvey Molotch. 2007. *Urban Fortunes: The Political Economy of Place*. Berkeley: University of California Press.

Long, Janet C., Frances C. Cunningham, and Jeffrey Bridges Braithwaite. 2013. "Brokers and Boundary Spanners in Collaborative Networks: A Systematic Review." *BMC Health Services Research* 13:158.

Lown Institute Hospitals Index. 2021. "Community Benefit." https://lownhospitalsindex.org/2021-winning-hospitals-community-benefit/. Accessed March 22, 2022.

Lurye, Rebecca 2021. "SINA's Latest Rehab Projects Are Building on Years of Resident-Driven Efforts to Fight Blight, Increase Home Ownership in Hartford." *Hartford Courant*, September 3.

Lusk, Katharine, and Monica Wang. 2019. "Enlisting America's Mayors as Public Health Allies." August 26. https://academyhealth.org/blog/2019-08/enlisting-americas-mayors-public-health-allies. Accessed December 27, 2022.

Luthi, Susannah. 2019. "Grassley Back at It, Ramping Up Scrutiny of Tax-Exempt Hospitals." *Modern Healthcare*, March 9. https://www.modernhealthcare.com/government/grassley-back-it-ramping-up-scrutiny-tax-exempt-hospitals. Accessed March 22, 2022.

MacDorman, Marian F., and Eugene Declercq. 2019. "Trends and State Variations in Out-of-Hospital Births in the United States, 2004–2017." *Birth* 46(2):279–88.

MacGillis, Alec. 2021. *Fulfillment: Winning and Losing in One-Click America*. New York: Farrar, Straus & Giroux.

Mailloux, Catherine, and E. Halesey. 2018. "Patient Navigators as Essential Members of the Healthcare Team: A Review of the Literature." *Journal of Nursing & Patient Care* 3:1.

Mannon, James M. 1976. Defining and Treating 'Problem Patients' in a Hospital Emergency Room." *Medical Care* 14(12):1004–13.

Marmot, Michael, and Richard Wilkinson, eds. 2005. *Social Determinants of Health.* Oxford: Oxford University Press.

Martin, Andrew. 2014. "State's Budget Cuts Hit the Young and Vulnerable." *Hartford Courant,* December 19.

Marwell, Nicole, and Michael McQuarrie. 2013. "People, Place, and System: Organizations and the Renewal of Urban Social Theory." *ANNALS of the American Academy of Political and Social Science* 647(1):126–43.

Massey, Douglas S., and Nancy A. Denton. 1998. *American Apartheid: Segregation and the Making of the Underclass.* Cambridge, MA: Harvard University Press.

Mayblin, Lucy, Gill Valentine, Florian Kossak, and Tatjana Schneider. 2015. "Experimenting with Spaces of Encounter: Creative Interventions to Develop Meaningful Contact." *Geoforum* 63:67–80.

McQuarrie, Michael. 2013. "Community Organizations in the Foreclosure Crisis: The Failure of Neoliberal Civil Society." *Politics & Society* 41(1):73–101.

Medical City Healthcare. n.d. "About Us." https://medicalcityhealthcare.com/about. Accessed January 22, 2022.

Meisel, Zachary, and Jesse Pines. 2008. "The Allure of the One-Stop Shop." *Slate.com,* September 12. https://slate.com/technology/2008/09/why-people-overuse-the-e-r.html. Accessed March 22, 2022.

Menchik, Daniel A. 2021. *Managing Medical Authority.* Princeton, NJ: University of Princeton Press.

Mettler, Suzanne. 2011. *The Submerged State: How Invisible Government Policies Undermine American Democracy.* Chicago: University of Chicago Press.

Metzl, Jonathan M., and Helena Hansen. 2014. "Structural Competency: Theorizing a New Medical Engagement with Stigma and Inequality." *Social Science & Medicine* 103:126–33.

Milken Institute. n.d. "Understanding Place-Based Philanthropy." https://milkeninstitute.org/article/understanding-place-based-philanthropy. Accessed February 25, 2022.

Minemeyer, Paige. 2016. "Hospitals Can Invest in Their Communities by Buying Locally." *Fierce Healthcare,* November 17. https://www.fiercehealthcare.com/healthcare/toolkit-encourage-hospitals-to-purchase-locally-sourced-goods. Accessed on September 4, 2021.

Minkler, Meredith, ed. 2012. *Community Organizing and Community Building for Health and Welfare,* 3rd ed. New Brunswick, NJ: Rutgers University Press.

Molotch, Harvey. 1976. "The City as a Growth Machine." *American Journal of Sociology* 82(2): 309–30.

Molotch, Harvey, William Freudenburg, and Krista E. Paulsen. 2000. "History Repeats Itself, But How? City Character, Urban Tradition, and the Accomplishment of Place." *American Sociological Review* 65(6):791–823.

Morse, Susan. 2015. "Healthcare Real Estate Deals Expected to Pick Up through 2015, Survey Says." *Healthcare Finance.* https://www.healthcarefinancenews.com/news/healthcare-real-estate-deals-expected-pick-through-2015-survey-says. Accessed September 4, 2021.

Murphy, John W. 2014. *Community-Based Interventions: Philosophy and Action.* New York: Springer.

Musumeci, MaryBeth, and Robin Rudowitz. 2016. "Medicaid Non-Emergency Medical Transportation: Overview and Key Issues in Medicaid Expansion Waivers." *KFF*, February 24.
https://www.kff.org/medicaid/issue-brief/medicaid-non-emergency-medical-transporta
tion-overview-and-key-issues-in-medicaid-expansion-waivers. Accessed March 22, 2022.

Nandyal, Samantha, David Strawhun, Hannah Stephen, Ashley Banks, and Daniel Skinner. 2021.
"Building Trust in American Hospital-Community Development Projects: A Scoping Review." *Journal of Community Hospital Internal Medicine Perspectives* 11:4:439–45.

Nápoles, Anna M., Jasmine Santoyo-Olsson, Leah S. Karliner, Steven E. Gregorich, and Eliseo J.
Pérez-Stable. 2015. "Inaccurate Language Interpretation and Its Clinical Significance in the
Medical Encounters of Spanish-Speaking Latinos." *Medical Care* 53(11):940–47.

Naramore, Floyd, William Bain Sr., Clifton Brady, and Perry Johanson. n.d. "The Cleveland
Clinic: Miller Family Pavilion and Glickman Tower." https://d3pxppq3195xue.cloudfront.net
/media/files/The_Cleveland_Clinic_nbbj_case_study_1.pdf. Accessed February 27, 2022.

Nassery, Najlla, Jodi B. Segal, Eva Chang, and John F. P. Bridges. 2015. "Systematic Overuse of Healthcare Services: A Conceptual Model." *Applied Health Economics and Health Policy* 13(1):1–6.

National Health Service. 2020. "Greener NHS Campaign to Tackle Climate 'Health Emergency.'"
January 5, 2020. https://www.england.nhs.uk/2020/01/greener-nhs-campaign-to-tackle-cli
mate-health-emergency/. Accessed December 21, 2022.

Nelson, Marla, and Laura Wolf-Powers. 2010. "Chains and Ladders: Exploring the Opportunities for Workforce Development and Poverty Reduction in the Hospital Sector." *Economic
Development Quarterly* 24(1):33–44.

Neubeck, Kenneth J., and Richard E. Ratcliff. 1988. "Urban Democracy and the Power of Corporate Capital: Struggles over Downtown Growth and Neighborhood Stagnation in Hartford,
Connecticut." In *Business Elites and Urban Development: Case Studies and Critical Perspectives*, ed. S. Cummings, 299–332. Albany: State University of New York Press.

NYU Langone Health. 2022. "City Health Dashboard." https://www.cityhealthdashboard.com/.
Accessed December 22, 2022.

O'Leary, Lizzie. 2020. "The Modern Supply Chain Is Snapping." *The Atlantic*, March 19.

Oliver, Carolyn. 2013. "Social Workers as Boundary Spanners: Reframing Our Professional Identity for Interprofessional Practice." *Social Work Education* 32(6):773–84.

Ollove, Michael. 2020. "Some Nonprofit Hospitals Aren't Earning Their Tax Breaks, Critics Say."
Stateline, February 7. https://www.pewtrusts.org/en/research-and-analysis/blogs/stateline/2020
/02/07/some-nonprofit-hospitals-arent-earning-their-tax-breaks-critics-say. Accessed December 22, 2022.

O'Reilly, Kevin B. 2020. "AMA: Racism Is a Threat to Public Health." November 16. https://www
.ama-assn.org/delivering-care/health-equity/ama-racism-threat-public-health. Accessed December 13, 2021.

Pager, Tyler, Lena H. Sun, and John Wagner. 2021. "Offering Beer, Babysitting and Barbershop
Outreach, the White House Launches New Initiatives to Boost Vaccinations." *Washington
Post,* June 2.

Papirno, Elissa. 1974. "Infant, Treated For Cold, Dies." *Hartford Courant*, March 27, p. 1.

Papirno, Elissa, and David Rhinelander. 1973. "City Care Decried in Tot's Death." *Hartford Courant*, January 20, p. 1.

Paremoer, Lauren, Sulakshana Nandi, Hani Serag, and Fran Baum. 2021. "Covid-19 Pandemic
and the Social Determinants of Health." *BMJ* 372. https://www.bmj.com/content/bmj/372
/bmj.n129.full.pdf. Accessed December 22, 2022.

Park, Sun Young, So Young Lee, and Yunan Chen. 2012. "The Effects of EMR Deployment on Doctors' Work Practices: A Qualitative Study in the Emergency Department of a Teaching Hospital." *International Journal of Medical Informatics* 81(3):204–17.

Parker, Charlie, Sam Scott, and Alistair Geddes. 2019. "Snowball Sampling." In *SAGE Research Methods Foundations*, ed. Paul Atkinson, Sara Delamont, Alexandru Cernat, Joseph W. Sakshaug, and Richard A. Williams. Thousand Oaks, CA: SAGE.

Patow, Carl, Debra Bryan, Gail Johnson, Eugenia Canaan, Adetolu Oyewo, Mukta Panda, Eric Walsh, and James Zaidan. 2016. "Who's in Our Neighborhood? Healthcare Disparities Experiential Education for Residents." *Ochsner Journal* 16(1):41–44.

Pattillo, Mary. 2007. *Black on the Block: The Politics of Race and Class in the City*. Chicago: University of Chicago Press.

Pease, Katherine. 2017. "Anchored in Place: How Funders Are Helping Anchor Institutions Strengthen Local Economies." Issue Lab, August 16. https://search.issuelab.org/resource /anchored-in-place-how-funders-are-helping-anchor-institutions-strengthen-local-econo mies.html. Accessed January 11, 2023.

Pennsylvania Department of State. 1997. "The Institutions of Purely Public Charity Act 10 P.S. § 371. et seq." https://www.dos.pa.gov/BusinessCharities/Charities/Resources/Pages/The -Institutions-of-Purely-Public-Charity-Act.aspx#.Vks9JU2FPq4. Accessed March 22, 2022.

Pescosolido, Bernice A. 1992. "Beyond Rational Choice: The Social Dynamics of How People Seek Help." *American Journal of Sociology* 97(4):1096–138.

Phelan, Jo C., and Bruce G. Link. 2015. "Is Racism a Fundamental Cause of Inequalities in Health?" *Annual Review of Sociology* 41(1):311–30.

Pollock, Rick. 2021. "Lown Institute Report on Hospital Community Benefits Falls Short." *American Hospital Association*, July 12. https://www.aha.org/news/blog/2021-07-12-lown -institute-report-hospital-community-benefits-falls-short. Accessed March 22, 2022.

Prakash, Mounika, and J. Carlton Johnny. 2015. "Things You Don't Learn in Medical School: Caduceus." *Journal of Pharmacy and Bioallied Sciences* 7 (Suppl 1.): S49–50.

Pratt, Mary Louise. 1991. "Arts of the Contact Zone." *Profession* 33–40.

Public Health Institute. 2017. "Increasing Transparency and Efficacy for Hospital Community Benefit Investments Nationwide." https://www.phi.org/about/impacts/increasing-trans parency-and-efficacy-for-hospital-community-benefit-investments-nationwide/. Accessed March 22, 2022.

Punski, Kevin 2018. "Mayo Clinic Ranked #1 Hospital in Florida by U.S. News and World Report." https://newsnetwork.mayoclinic.org/discussion/mayo-clinic-ranked-no-1-hospital-in -florida-by-u-s-news-world-report/. Accessed March 22, 2022.

Quadagno, Jill. 2000. "Promoting Civil Rights through the Welfare State: How Medicare Integrated Southern Hospitals." *Social Problems* 47(1):68–89.

Ravi, Rao, Hawkins Melissa, Ulrich Trina, Gatlin Greta, Mabry Guadalupe, and Mishra Chaitanya. 2020. "The Evolving Role of Public Health in Medical Education." *Frontiers in Public Health* 8. https://www.frontiersin.org/articles/10.3389/fpubh.2020.00251

Raudenbush, Danielle T. 2020. *Health Care Off the Books: Poverty, Illness, and Strategies for Survival in Urban America*. Berkeley: University of California Press.

Reich, Jennifer. 2016. *Calling the Shots*. New York: NYU Press.

Releford, Bill J., Stanley K. Frencher Jr., and Antronette K. Yancey. 2010. "Health Promotion in Barbershops: Balancing Outreach and Research in African American Communities." *Ethnicity & Disease* 20(2):185–88.

Reynolds, Preston P. 1997. "The Federal Government's Use of Title VI and Medicare to Racially Integrate Hospitals in the United States, 1963 through 1967." *American Journal of Public Health* 87(11):1850–58.

Rhomberg, Chris. 2007. *No There There: Race, Class, and Political Community in Oakland.* Berkeley: University of California Press.

Rice, Joseph D. 1979. "Therapy Center Might Wipe Out Willis' Businesses on Euclid Avenue." *The Plain Dealer,* August 21.

Richter, Andreas W., Michael A. West, Rolf van Dick, and Jeremy F. Dawson. 2017. "Boundary Spanners' Identification, Intergroup Contact, and Effective Intergroup Relations." *Academy of Management Journal* 49(6):1252–69.

Rienzi, Greg. 2013. "The Changing Face of East Baltimore." *Johns Hopkins University Gazette,* January. https://hub.jhu.edu/gazette/2013/january/east-baltimore-changes-development/. Accessed December 22, 2022.

Robbins, Blaine G. 2012. "A Blessing and a Curse? Political Institutions in the Growth and Decay of Generalized Trust: A Cross-National Panel Analysis, 1980–2009." *PLoS ONE* 7(4):e35120.

Roberts, Michael. 2019. "Denver's Ten Most Dangerous Intersections." *Westword,* June 17. https://www.westword.com/news/denver-most-dangerous-intersections-now-13680355. Accessed December 22, 2022.

Rojas, Reinaldo. 2015. "Community Development and Its Socioeconomic Impact on a Latino Enclave: A Case Study of the Frog Hollow Neighborhood in Hartford, Connecticut." Doctoral diss., University of Connecticut, August 10.

Romano, Max J. 2018. "White Privilege in a White Coat: How Racism Shaped My Medical Education." *Annals of Family Medicine* 16(3):261–63.

Rosenbaum, Sara. 2013. "The Enduring Role of the Emergency Medical Treatment and Active Labor Act." *Health Affairs* 32(12):2075–81.

Rosenbaum, Sara, Amber Rieke, and Maureen Byrnes. 2014. "Encouraging Nonprofit Hospitals to Invest in Community Building: The Role Of IRS 'Safe Harbors.'" *Health Affairs Blog,* February 11. https://www.healthaffairs.org/do/10.1377/hblog20140211.037060/full/. Accessed March 22, 2022.

Rosenberg, Charles E. 1987. *The Care of Strangers: The Rise of America's Hospital System.* New York: Basic Books.

Rosner, David. 1982. *A Once Charitable Enterprise: Hospitals and Health Care in Brooklyn and New York, 1885–1915,* Cambridge: Cambridge University Press.

Ross, Tracey. 2014. "Eds, Meds, and the Feds." Center for American Progress, October 24. https://www.americanprogress.org/article/eds-meds-and-the-feds/.

Rothkopf, David. 2009. *Superclass.* New York: Farrar, Straus & Giroux.

Rothstein, Richard. 2017. *The Color of Law: A Forgotten History of How Our Government Segregated America.* New York: Liveright.

Rubin, Daniel B., Simone R. Singh, and Gary J. Young. 2015. "Tax-Exempt Hospitals and Community Benefit: New Directions in Policy and Practice." *Annual Review of Public Health* 36(1):545–57.

Sampson, Robert J. 1991. "Linking the Micro and the Macrolevel Dimensions of Community Social Organization." *Social Forces* 70:43–64.

———. 2012. *Great American City: Chicago and the Enduring Neighborhood Effect.* Chicago: University of Chicago Press.

———. 2019. "Neighbourhood Effects and Beyond: Explaining the Paradoxes of Inequality in the Changing American Metropolis." *Urban Studies* 56(1):3–32.

Sanborn, Beth J. 2017. "IRS Revokes Tax-Exempt Status for County-Run Hospital, Raising Specter of More Actions against Nonprofits." *Healthcare Finance News*, August 16. https://www.healthcarefinancenews.com/news/irs-revokes-tax-exempt-status-county-run-hospital-raising-specter-more-actions-against. Accessed March 22, 2022.

Sanger-Katz, Margot. 2019. "Warren Has Her Plan. Buttigieg Suggests Another Way to Cut Health Prices." *New York Times*, November 6. https://www.nytimes.com/2019/11/06/upshot/buttigieg-health-care-plan.html.

Schensul, Stephen L., Maria Borrero, Victoria Barrera, Jeffrey Backstrand, and Peter Guarnaccia. 1982. "A Model of Fertility Control in a Puerto Rican Community." *Urban Anthropology* 11(1):81–99.

Schiller, Zach. 2018. "Local Tax Abatement in Ohio: A Flash of Transparency." January 18. https://www.policymattersohio.org/research-policy/quality-ohio/revenue-budget/tax-policy/local-tax-abatement-in-ohio-a-flash-of-transparency. Accessed December 8, 2021.

Schoenberg, Sandra Perlman. 1980. "Some Trends in the Community Participation of Women in Their Neighborhoods." *Signs* 5(3):263–68.

Schorch, Philipp. 2013. "Contact Zones, Third Spaces, and the Act of Interpretation." *Museum and Society* 11:68–81.

Schnoke, Molly, Merissa Piazza, Heather Smith, and Liam Robinson. 2018. "Greater University Circle Initiative: Year 7 Evaluation Report." *Urban Publications*. https://engagedscholarship.csuohio.edu/urban_facpub/1548. Accessed March 22, 2022.

Schumacher, Patrick, and Leigh Wedenoja. 2022. "Home or Hospital: What Place of Death Can Tell Us about COVID-19 and Public Health." Rockefeller Institute of Government (blog), June 2. https://rockinst.org/blog/home-or-hospital-what-place-of-death-can-tell-us-about-covid-19-and-public-health/. Accessed December 21, 2022.

Scott, W. Richard, Martin Ruef, Peter J. Mendel, and Carol A. Caronna. 2000. *Institutional Change and Healthcare Organizations: From Professional Dominance to Managed Care*. Chicago: University of Chicago Press.

Scruggs, Afi. 2020. "A Quarter of Cuyahoga County Homes Have No Internet Access—Why That Matters and How It's Changing." *Cleveland.com*, February 26. https://www.cleveland.com/news/2020/02/a-quarter-of-cuyahoga-county-homes-have-no-internet-access-why-that-matters-and-how-its-changing.html. Accessed September 6, 2021.

Security Magazine. 2011. "Advancing the University of Colorado Hospital's Security Program." https://www.securitymagazine.com/articles/82456-advancing-the-university-of-colorado-hospitals-security-program. Accessed November 19, 2021.

Seim, Josh 2020. *Bandage, Sort, and Hustle: Ambulance Crews on the Front Lines of Urban Suffering*. Berkeley: University of California Press.

The Sentinel. 2015. "Community Compassion Funds Aurora Man's Miraculous Recovery." *The Sentinel*, August 12. https://sentinelcolorado.com/news/community-compassion-funds-aurora-mans-miraculous-recovery.

Sharkey, Patrick. 2013. *Stuck in Place: Urban Neighborhoods and the End of Progress Toward Racial Equality*. Chicago: University of Chicago Press.

Shils, Edward. 1975. *Center and Periphery: Essays in Macrosociology*. Chicago and London: University of Chicago Press.

Shortell, Stephen M., Robin R. Gillies, and Kelly J. Devers. 1995. "Reinventing the American Hospital." *Milbank Quarterly* 73(2):131–60.

Silverberg, Jay. 2016. "The New Academic Hybrid: Creating a Mixed-Use Campus Community." Spaces4Learning. https://spaces4learning.com/articles/2016/10/01/academic-hybrid.aspx. Accessed March 22, 2022.

Singer, Merrill. 2003. "An Organizational Life Cycle Perspective on the Development of the Hispanic Health Council." *Practicing Anthropology* 25(3):46–51.

Skinner, Daniel, Janelle Donovan-Lyle, and Kelly J. Kelleher. 2014. "Housing and Child Health: Safety Net Strategies, Regulations and Neighborhood Challenges." *Journal of Applied Research on Children* 5(2).

Skinner, Daniel, Berkeley Franz, and Kelly Kelleher. 2018. "What Challenges Do Appalachian Non-Profit Hospitals Face in Taking on Community Health Needs Assessments? A Qualitative Study from Ohio." *Journal of Rural Health* 34(2):182–92.

Skinner, Daniel, Berkeley Franz, Robert Penfold, and Kelly Kelleher. 2018. "Community Perceptions of Hospitals and Shared Physical Space: A Qualitative Study." *Culture, Medicine, and Psychiatry* 42(1):131–58.

Skinner, Daniel, William Gardner, and Kelly Kelleher. 2016. "When Hospitals Join the Community: Practical Considerations and Ethical Frameworks." *Journal of Health Care for the Poor and Underserved* 27(3):1171–82.

Skloot, Rebecca. 2010. *The Immortal Life of Henrietta Lacks*. New York: Crown Publishers.

Sloan, Frank A. 1980. "The Internal Organization of Hospitals: A Descriptive Study." *Health Services Research* 15(3):203–30.

Small, Mario Luis. 2004. *Villa Victoria: The Transformation of Social Capital in a Boston Barrio*. Chicago: University of Chicago Press.

———. 2006. "Neighborhood Institutions as Resource Brokers: Childcare Centers, Interorganizational Ties, and Resource Access among the Poor." *Social Problems* 53(2):274–92.

Solomon, Loel S., and Michael H. Kanter. 2018. "Health Care Steps Up to Social Determinants of Health: Current Context." *The Permanente Journal* 22:18–139.

Somerville, Martha H., Laura Seeff, Daniel Hale, and Daniel J. O'Brien. 2015. "Hospitals, Collaboration, and Community Health Improvement." *Journal of Law, Medicine & Ethics* 43(S1):56–59.

Song, Ji Seon. 2021. "Policing the Emergency Room." *Harvard Law Review* 134(8):2646–720.

Spiro, Ellen. 1990. *DiAna's Hair Ego*. Women Make Movies and Video Data Bank.

Stainback, Kevin, Donald Tomaskovic-Devey, and Sheryl Skaggs. 2010. "Organizational Approaches to Inequality: Inertia, Relative Power, and Environments." *Annual Review of Sociology* 36:1:225–47.

Starr, Paul. 1982. *The Social Transformation of American Medicine*. New York: Basic Books.

Steadman, Henry J. 1992. "Boundary Spanners: A Key Component for the Effective Interactions of the Justice and Mental Health Systems." *Law and Human Behavior* 16:75–87.

Stefanowicz, Michael, Brett Feldman, and Jehni Robinson. 2021. "House Calls Without Walls: Street Medicine Delivers Primary Care to Unsheltered Persons Experiencing Homelessness." *Annals of Family Medicine* 19(1):84.

Stevens, Rosemary. 1989. *In Sickness and in Wealth: American Hospitals in the Twentieth Century*. New York: Basic Books.

Stinchcombe, Arthur. 1968. *Constructing Social Theories*. Chicago: University of Chicago Press.

Stone, Ashley, Debby Rogers, Sheree Kruckenberg, and Alexis Lieser. 2012. "Impact of the Mental Healthcare Delivery System on California Emergency Departments." *Western Journal of Emergency Medicine* 13(1):51–56.

Stowe, Stacey. 2000. "Raising the Neighborhood." *New York Times*, October 29, p.14.

Subica, Andrew M., and Bruce G. Link. 2022. "Cultural Traumas as Fundamental Cause of Health Disparities." *Social Science & Medicine* 292:e114574.

Sullivan, Kevin B., and James A. Trostle. 2004. "Trinity College and the Learning Corridor: A Small, Urban Liberal Arts College Launches a Public Magnet School Campus." *Metropolitan Universities* 15(3):15–34.

Tarraf, Wassim, William Vega, and Hector M. González. 2014. "Emergency Department Services Use among Immigrant and Non-Immigrant Groups in the United States." *Journal of Immigrant and Minority Health* 16(4):595–606.

Taylor, Lauren. 2018. "Housing and Health: An Overview of the Literature." *Health Affairs Health Policy Brief*, June 7. https://www.healthaffairs.org/do/10.1377/hpb20180313.396577/full/. Accessed December 13, 2021.

Thompson, John D., and Grace Goldin. 1975. *The Hospital: A Social and Architectural History.* New Haven, CT: Yale University Press.

Tozzi, John. 2021. "Medical Debt Is Crushing Black Americans, and Hospitals Aren't Helping." *Bloomberg Businessweek*, November 22. https://www.bloomberg.com/news/features /2021-11-22/medical-debt-collection-tactics-disproportionately-hit-black-americans. Accessed March 22, 2022.

Trickey, Erick. 2003. "A Palace Away from Home." *Cleveland Magazine,* January 1. https://cleveland magazine.com/in-the-cle/people/articles/a-palace-away-from-home. Accessed March 22, 2022.

Tringer, Grant. 2017. "After Housing Crisis, Aurora Using Pot Funds to Resettle Motel Residents." *Westword*, September 19. https://www.westword.com/news/aurora-resettles-kings -inn-motel-residents-with-pot-tax-funds-9498028. Accessed December 13, 2021.

UCHealth. 2019a. "University of Colorado Hospital Community Health Needs Assessment." https://uchealth-wp-uploads.s3.amazonaws.com/wp-content/uploads/2019/06/19104746 /ABOUT-UCHealth-UCH-2019-CHNA-Report.pdf. Accessed October 18, 2022.

———. 2019b. "University of Colorado Hospital Implementation Strategy." https://uchealth-wp -uploads.s3.amazonaws.com/wp-content/uploads/2019/10/24083918/ABOUT-UCHealth -UCH-CHNA-2019-Implementation-Strategy-Report.pdf. Accessed October 18, 2022.

United Nations. 2019. "World Economic Situation and Prospects." https://www.un.org/devel-opment/desa/dpad/wp-content/uploads/sites/45/WESP2019_BOOK-ANNEX-en.pdf. Accessed February 20, 2022.

University of Colorado Anschutz Medical Campus. 2021. "2021 Annual Security and Fire Safety Report." https://www.cuanschutz.edu/docs/librariesprovider37/default-document-library/2021 -final-cu-anschutz-annual-security-reporte8dcb0e6302864d9a5bfff0a001ce385.pdf?Status =Temp&sfvrsn=27f4d4ba_2. Accessed February 20, 2022.

U.S. Department of Education. 2016. "The Handbook for Campus Safety and Security Reporting 2016 Edition." https://www2.ed.gov/admins/lead/safety/handbook.pdf. Accessed December 22, 2022.

U.S. Department of Health and Human Services. 2017. "Sex, Race, and Ethnic Diversity of U.S. Health Occupations (2011–2015)." https://bhw.hrsa.gov/sites/default/files/bureau-health -workforce/data-research/diversity-us-health-occupations.pdf. Accessed December 13, 2021.

————. n.d. "Social Determinants of Health." Healthy People 2030. https://health.gov/healthy people/objectives-and-data/social-determinants-health. Accessed February 3, 2022.

U.S. General Accountability Office. 2020. "Tax Administration: Opportunities Exist to Improve Oversight of Hospitals Tax-Exempt Status." https://www.gao.gov/products/gao-20-679. Accessed December 12, 2021.

van Ham, Maarten, and David Manley. 2012. "Neighbourhood Effects Research at a Crossroads: Ten Challenges for Future Research Introduction." *Environment and Planning A: Economy and Space* 44(12):2787–93.

Verderber, Stephen. 2010. *Innovations in Hospital Architecture*. London: Routledge.

Verghese, Abraham. 2012. *Cutting for Stone: A Novel*. London: Random House.

von Hoffman, Alexander. 2013. "The Past, Present, and Future of Community Development." *Shelterforce*. https://shelterforce.org/2013/07/17/the_past_present_and_future_of_community _development/. Accessed September 4, 2021.

Wacquant, Loïc. 2008. *Urban Outcasts: A Comparative Sociology of Advanced Marginality*. Malden, MA: Polity.

————. 2009. *Punishing the Poor: The Neoliberal Government of Social Insecurity*. Durham, NC, and London: Duke University Press.

Wacquant, Loïc, and William J. Wilson. 1989. "The Cost of Racial and Class Exclusion in the Inner City." *Annals of the American Academy of Political and Social Science* 501:8–25.

Watkins-Hayes, Celeste. 2009. "Race-Ing the Bootstrap Climb: Black and Latino Bureaucrats in Post-Reform Welfare Offices." *Social Problems* 56(2):285–310.

Weber, Natalie. 2018. "Aurora Embraces Role as the Top Landing Spot for Immigrants in Colorado." *Denver Post*, July 15.

Weil, Thomas P. 2012. "Why Are ACOs Doomed for Failure?" *Journal of Medical Practice Management* 27(5):263–67.

Weiss, Audrey J., Lauren M. Wier, and Carol Stocks, et al. 2006. Overview of Emergency Department Visits in the United States, 2011: Statistical Brief #174. 2014 Jun. In Healthcare Cost and Utilization Project (HCUP) Statistical Briefs [Internet]. Rockville (MD): Agency for Healthcare Research and Quality (US); 2006 Feb.

Weyeneth, Robert R. 2001. "The Power of Apology and the Process of Historical Reconciliation." *The Public Historian* 23(3):9–38.

Wherry, Frederick. 2010. "Producing the Character of Place." *Journal of Urban History* 36(4):554–60.

Wiley, Chelsea. n.d. "Say Goodbye to Mount Carmel West: The Hospital Will Be Demolished Spring 2019." *Columbus Navigator*. https://www.columbusnavigator.com/say-goodbye-mount-car mel-west-hospital-will-demolished-spring. Accessed March 27, 2022.

Willis-Carrasco, Aundra. n.d. "The Jazz Temple." *Cleveland Historical*. https://clevelandhistori cal.org/items/show/811. Accessed February 2, 2022.

Wilson, Helen F. 2011. "Passing Propinquities in the Multicultural City: The Everyday Encounters of Bus Passengering." *Environment and Planning: Economy and Space* 43:634–49.

Wilson, Robert N. 1963. "The Social Structure of a General Hospital." *Annals of the American Academy of Political and Social Science* 346(1):67–76.

Wilson, William Julius. 1987. *The Truly Disadvantaged: The Inner City, the Underclass, and Public Policy*. Chicago: University of Chicago Press.

Winant, Gabriel. 2021. *The Next Shift: The Fall of Industry and the Rise of Health Care in Rust Belt America*. Chicago: University of Chicago Press.

Wyland, Michael. 2013. "Avoiding Misconceptions in Filing Community Health Needs Assessments." *Non-Profit Quarterly*, March 12. https://nonprofitquarterly.org/avoiding-misconceptions-in-filing-community-health-needs-assessments/. Accessed March 22, 2022.

———. 2017. "Hospital Loses IRS Tax Exemption for Noncompliance with ACA." *Non-Profit Quarterly*, August 18. https://nonprofitquarterly.org/hospital-loses-irs-tax-exemption. Accessed March 24, 2022.

Wynn, Jonathan R. 2015. *Music/City: American Festivals and Placemaking in Austin, Nashville, and Newport.* Chicago: University of Chicago Press.

Young, Gary J., Chia-Hung Chou, Jeffrey Alexander, Shoou-Yih Daniel Lee, and Eli Raver. 2013. "Provision of Community Benefits by Tax-Exempt U.S. Hospitals." *New England Journal of Medicine* 368:1519–27.

Young, Kathryn, and Katie Billings. 2020. "Legal Consciousness and Cultural Capital." *Law & Society Review* 54(1):33–65.

Zeuli, Kimberly. 2015. "New Incentives and Opportunities for Hospitals to Engage in Local Economic Development." *Economic Development Journal* 14(1):20–28.

Zhou, Min. 1993. *Chinatown: The Socioeconomic Potential of an Urban Enclave.* Philadelphia: Temple University Press.

Index

Printed and bound by CPI Group (UK) Ltd, Croydon, CR0 4YY

09/06/2025

14685759-0001